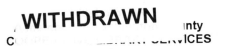

CHRONICALLY
Fabulous

CHRONICALLY
Fabulous

FINDING **WHOLENESS** AND **HOPE** LIVING WITH CHRONIC ILLNESS

Marisa Zeppieri

 Broadleaf Books

Minneapolis

Dad,
May we see each other in eternity,
to spend the time we missed here on earth.

Contents

1 Wrong Place, Wrong Time   1

2 A Heaping Serving of Love   11

3 Seeing Potential—Even in the Fight of Your Life   23

4 A Lesson in Silence   41

5 Timelines and Triggers   59

6 Seasons of Recalibration   79

7 Our Uniquely Designed Purpose   95

8 Use Your Voice—Even If It Shakes   105

9 A Fortress Made of True Friends   121

10 Flares, Frankfurters, and Other Catastrophes   137

11 The Heat of the Fire   149

12 My Kitchen, My Situation Room   161

13 Speak All of Your Truth   177

14 What It Means to Be Made Whole   187

Notes   197

ONE

Wrong Place,
Wrong Time

There are two kinds of pain in this world:
pain that hurts, and pain that alters.
—Denzel Washington

When I was twenty-two years old, taking an afternoon stroll in North Miami's Aventura Mall, a raven-haired elderly lady veered past a small crowd and made her way over to me. Everything about her radiated *free spirit*: a colorful headscarf, a flowing dress with multiple layers of lace, and long, vibrant, jeweled necklaces that danced around her upper body as she moved. I was startled when she stopped directly in front of me and looked me in the eyes. Gently taking my hands, she said, "God will use these hands to change people's lives." She made the visionary statement with complete certainty.

Today when I think about that moment, I realize I never answered her. In my surprise at her unbidden declaration, I could only stare into her deep caramel-colored eyes and nod my head up and down in appeasing agreement. Though it seemed like a random event at first, I couldn't stop thinking about this woman and what she said as I drove back home that day.

At the time, I was already several years into a college program to earn my registered nursing degree. I had a life plan. This plan was on a schedule and offered me stability, financial freedom, and a meaningful outlet for one of my greatest passions—helping people.

Nursing checked all the boxes. Sure, I would use my hands to hang IVs, deliver medication, and offer someone comfort by holding theirs during a challenging moment or eternal transition, but my gut told me this stranger's message held a deeper meaning—that my hands would be used to provide guidance and comfort in a way that didn't involve nursing.

The moment of meeting her was striking, though after years passed, I forgot the message and the messenger. Coming out of a season of complete brokenness, the life plan I had so meticulously created ended in a set of unforgettable moments. And instead of becoming a nurse and working in the medical field to save the lives of others, it took an extraordinary team of nurses and medical personnel to save my own life.

Now that one sentence spoken to me by a complete stranger took on an entirely different meaning for my life.

What began as a day of errands and work on a breathtaking April Sunday in 2001 ended in my fight for survival. Two events lined up at the exact moment on that day: a drunk driver (also under the influence of drugs) in a pickup truck and me, a pedestrian, barely weighing in at one hundred pounds, crossing a street. And for reasons I believe are far greater than we humans can understand, my body and the frame of that Ford Ranger traveling around forty-five miles per hour collided just after 7 p.m. in downtown Fort Lauderdale.

One drunk driver on drugs.

One truck.

One moment.

That is all it took to forever alter the course of my life. To crush my body. And to rip me away from the dreams and goals that fueled my waking hours—and the independence I sought.

The event broke me in every way you can possibly imagine. During my yearlong recovery, and for some time after, I dealt with the impact of that single moment, physically overcoming broken ribs, internal bleeding, a fractured pelvis, a multilacerated liver, and a head injury. The cumulative impact required months of rehab for me to begin walking again. Emotionally, the struggle continued well beyond the many grueling daily hours of rehab as feelings of frustration, bitterness, anger, and depression took hold. I daily battled PTSD, and spiritually, I was on a desperate search for answers.

Why did this happen?

Why did I survive?

How did I survive?

And how *will* I move forward?

As I watched so much of my hard work and many of my dreams come to an unexpected and abrupt end, I questioned whether there could be something bigger than myself at work.

Many of us experience seasons of brokenness in our lives. Yours may not have been triggered by three thousand pounds of steel barreling toward you, but the impact was likely just as crushing, just as traumatic. Life will hit us with different seasons that knock us to the ground, leaving us battered, bruised, and feeling empty.

No one is exempt.

We battle with illness and loneliness, divorce, death of our loved ones, our identity, infertility, financial ruin, accidents, and chronic illness, as well as other challenges that are societal, environmental. Life's trials often leave us with mascara-stained cheeks and swollen lips, our faces buried in our bedroom pillows. In that brokenness, we often feel completely helpless. And it can be hard to recognize in the midst of this brokenness that what we do in these moments, when the world seems dark and we feel completely alone, will shape our beliefs and ultimately our legacy.

Unlike other difficult times, this season of brokenness was one of the most difficult I ever faced, and it brought me to the end of myself. And it may sound odd, but it's also something for which I am eternally grateful. Coming to the end of myself forced me to purge self-sufficiency and recognize that something much greater than myself was at work in my life. It turned my young mind from being obsessed with life planning and a career and directed it toward a higher purpose.

That fateful April day, I found myself suddenly trapped. Anger and bitterness began to take root; crippling, PTSD-fueled anxiety attacks spawned out of nowhere. Losing my independence and having to solely rely on others because of the physical injuries I endured put me over the edge.

And that also became the start of my struggle with severe autoimmune issues.

While many have different ways they consider and depend on a higher power, for me, the situation led me to turn to my faith tradition. In Psalms, there's a reference to God's response to those who have a "broken spirit" (Psalm 51:17). This isn't a reference to our being shamed or degraded or beaten down—but as I read it and relate it to my life, it refers to a sense of God witnessing that moment of my life where my own spirit reached the end of itself. In that moment and in my desperation to be free, I discovered God—a God who wouldn't leave me in a broken state. A God who does great work from broken places, slowly restoring and rebuilding us.

It's in this moment where our independence and self-reliance have been released that the rebuilding process can begin.

I was desperate to be nourished and rebuilt. My body was physically unrecognizable, but a deep kind of joy and excitement began to manifest as each new day now brought unrecognized challenges. Years later, I understood that this season in my life—from the moment of impact to rehab to the longer challenge of immune issues—was an opportunity to grow and discover God working in me.

A new hunger began to emerge. I discovered an insatiable emotional, spiritual, and physical hunger. And I devoured the learning process, discovering knowledge in a variety of areas—food, nutrition, medicine, the Bible, and learning around God-given gifts and a life of purpose.

Through the mentoring of my gastronomically gifted Italian grandmother, I learned how to nourish my broken body with the help of food and herbs. She also helped me discover that

Fabulous Finds

Name Your Role Models and Supporters

Take a few moments and jot down the names of those who have served as role models, supporters, and cheerleaders during your most challenging seasons. Write a note to or take a few minutes to call these special people and thank them for their encouragement and love.

my broken heart, my ended dreams, and my crushed spirit were a starting place to learn faith.

As I started writing this book, I began to see that so much of the wisdom of food, of nutrition, of faith was shared with me by my grandmother and my mother—two women who had a monumental impact on my life and my recovery.

All of us, I'd wager, while our life stories are different, have key figures who served as role models, wisdom givers, and comforters. Sometimes it takes some deeper reflection to surface those names. But holding fast to your memories of these special people, even as you read this book, may help you rediscover and awaken some life-shifting advice or experience you may have tucked away that now can help guide you through your current challenges.

My hope is that by sharing my stories and the insights I have gained about rebuilding a life, releasing psychological brokenness, living in hope, and discovering nutrition and the healing ways of food, I can encourage you to persevere through your own difficult seasons, your loss or silence or mourning. You may experience the outside world as cold, barren, and winter-like. But my hope is that through this book, you will remember that even if loss or a chronic condition makes you feel broken, spring is just around the corner.

Your season *is* going to change.

And spring is a time of planting, rebuilding, and regrowth. Spring, as I reflect on it, is the season of the seed, the season of something so powerful and small—small enough that if we saw it on the sidewalk or on a table, we would ignore it or brush it off. But the thing about a seed is that it has to be immersed into sudden darkness, it has to break open first so that it can grow. So that like a seedling with a unique identity and design, it allows that which is greater than you—perhaps the thing you call the ground of all being, God—to work in you when you are buried deep in total darkness, preparing you to push your way through hardened, brutal ground in order to allow the light of God to nourish you and provide the sustenance you need to live out your wonderful purpose.

There's a profound connection I have discovered on this journey through brokenness and restoration. And a link between faith and food—how they both hold the incredible power to heal, nourish, and rebuild our lives.

Whatever challenge has brought you to this book, I hope you'll discover that even what is chronic or broken and waiting to emerge can be fabulous, whole, life-giving—and lifesaving. Especially you.

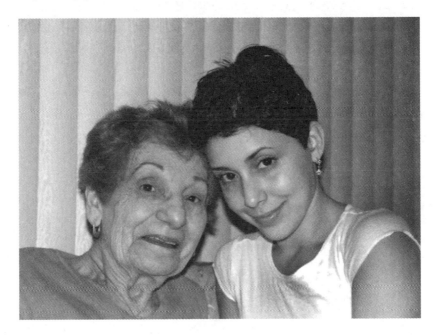

Carrot, Ginger, and Turmeric Soup with Orange

Prep Time: 15 minutes
Cook Time: 30–35 minutes
Method: Stovetop, blender, or immersion blender
Yield: 4–6 servings

Sometimes we are overwhelmed and can't eat anything. Sometimes all we want is something nourishing. To me, there is nothing better than a warm, creamy soup on a chilly fall or winter evening. Made with fresh ginger and turmeric, this recipe packs a lot of anti-inflammatory power behind it while also nourishing your body with a variety of nutrients. Plus, the cayenne and black pepper (I add extra) give this soup a deep, peppery undertone. If you don't have butternut squash on hand, you can use extra carrots. And there are many ways to add a final touch depending on your tastes, such as topping it off with plain Greek yogurt, parsley, or even spicy chopped jalapeños. Enjoy!

INGREDIENTS

2 tablespoons olive oil
2 cups carrots, chopped
2 cups butternut squash, chopped
1 yellow onion, chopped
1 fennel bulb, greens removed, chopped
4 cloves garlic, pressed or minced
2–3-inch nub of fresh ginger, grated
1 tablespoon turmeric
¼ teaspoon Himalayan or sea salt
¼–½ teaspoon black pepper (depending on your preference)
Dash or two of cayenne pepper
3 cups vegetable broth
½ cup milk or milk alternative
Zest of 1 medium orange

Optional Toppings
Fresh parsley
Plain Greek yogurt
Minced jalapeños
Cracked black pepper
Extra salt
Cumin
Avocado

In a large saucepan or Dutch oven, heat oil on medium to high heat. Add carrots, butternut squash, onion, and fennel. Sauté until the vegetables start to soften, about 5 minutes. Add garlic, ginger, turmeric, salt, pepper, and cayenne to the saucepan and cook for another 3 minutes or so. Next, add vegetable broth, milk or milk alternative, and orange zest. Bring all of this to a boil, then cover and simmer the mixture for about 20 minutes.

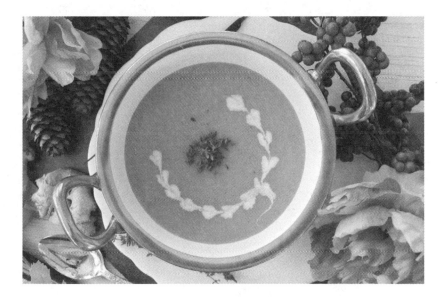

Turn off heat and let the soup sit for about five minutes. Next, add the soup to a blender in batches, blending each batch for a few seconds until creamy. An easier method for this step is using an immersion blender directly in the saucepan. Once the entire soup has been blended, add additional salt and pepper to your taste preference. Serve immediately. You can top this soup off with Greek yogurt, parsley, or even avocado!

TWO

A Heaping Serving
of Love

You don't choose your family. They are
God's gift to you, as you are to them.
—Desmond Tutu

Saturdays were reserved for baking in my grandmother's kitchen. Everyone waited in anticipation all week long, praying biscotti, pignoli cookies, and chocolate-filled rugelach would be on the menu. In true Italian custom, we found my grandmother in the kitchen each morning by 6:30 a.m. formulating the day's culinary endeavors.

Like most Italian families and many cultures, cuisine—its preparation and delivery into as many mouths as humanly possible—has always been an integral part of our family's life. But for my grandmother, the kitchen was her sanctuary. And unless a family member was specifically invited in, it was common knowledge in my family that you stayed out of her way. If a child crossed the threshold, a wooden spoon might threaten, or if an adult entered and interrupted the process, there was usually a naughty word or two in Italian headed their way.

The off-limits rules of my grandmother's kitchen sanctuary had only one exception: *me.*

I can't tell you if she was tickled by my fascination for cooking or if she noticed a creative talent for food I was still too young to comprehend, but I quickly became her trusted kitchen sidekick. She was eager to pour out knowledge about her intimate, healing relationship with food, and I drank it all in. And in her own stoic way, she was eager to pour out love, which I fully consumed.

For me, the kitchen held a kind of sacred light, a healing light. Those lights were ones I would later return to, peruse like a shelf of healing spices and herbs, each moment with its own wisdom or scent of love and support. The light of my grandmother shined in those thousands of hours we spent together in her kitchen. When I needed that support most, the reminder that I am loved, and that I was safe, that light was there. And the memories of a healing kitchen continue to be a stabilizing force for me when life events dim that light. It's those distinctive life moments all of us have met that we can hold deeply in our memory—where unconditional love and hope reside. Those memories continually remind us of the healing people and healing spaces we were blessed by, memories that can still bring us balance and peace during troubled times.

When I was a child, I didn't quite understand how significant a role the kitchen would play throughout my entire life. But it grew in its significance, even in my childhood. Becoming comfortable in the kitchen was my first challenge. At the start, my grandmother delegated the simplest of tasks to me. For a lengthy season, I was the flour girl. It was my job to evenly and lightly dust flour all over her round glass tabletop in the corner of her small, gold-and-avocado-colored kitchen. My young, tiny hands could only hold so much flour. But where I fell short in speed, I made up with an intense desire to be precise. *Am I going too slow?* I wondered as I meticulously spread the flour. But she never rushed me. Instead, she was a continuous source of encouragement, nodding her head in acknowledgment of a job well done, followed by an exuberant "You're getting better every day!" Once my task was complete, a fine dusting of flour not only covered the tabletop but lingered in a heavy cloud in the air. My grandmother would position a thick slab of dough on top of the table and get to work.

Tiny and barely weighing a hundred pounds, my grandmother Rose was a powerhouse. And what she lacked in size, she made up for in wit, talent, wisdom, and a fiery personality. We often called her "The General," "Chief," or "Sarge."

Not everyone has a "Rose" or a "Chief" in their life, maybe not a grandmother or even a relative. But perhaps a mentor or friend, a confidant, cooking buddy, or secret-keeper has been a steady presence in your life, someone you've seen as a gift. These gift mentors are those who see the best and the worst in us and continue to love us just the same. I've been blessed to have life-giving, God-given relationships early in life with both my grandmother and my mother by my side.

And for me, that bond with my grandmother was heightened and amplified through our mutual love for the kitchen and creating culinary masterpieces for our family to enjoy.

As I matured in those early years, more tasks were added to my proverbial plate. Although I was only allowed to watch her work her magic in the kitchen (aside from flour dusting), I was later given responsibility for preparing the mise en place. When I was eight years old, my favorite recipe to create with Grandma was the rugelach. Grandma adapted her own recipe after years of sampling pastries from Jewish neighbors while growing up in East New York. While not an Italian baked good, the Ashke-nazic pastry was her favorite and topped our Saturday-morning kitchen to-do list. The filling would also be different, however. Some weeks it was chocolate, and other weeks a combination of raisins, preserves, cinnamon, and walnuts.

My grandmother would stand closely behind me, wrapping her arms around mine. The scent of her perfume, a warm vanilla musk, filled the air, while out of the corner of my eye I would catch glimpses of auburn-colored waves framing her face. Gently cupping her hands over mine, we would lift the wide side of the triangular piece of dough together and roll it to form the crescent-shaped rugelach.

"Try to keep the dough tight, Marisa," Grandma gently reminded me as we slowly rolled an individual piece of rugelach. "We don't want any of those goodies falling out," she added, a wink in her eye as she stepped away, allowing me a solo attempt.

At first, the triangles I shaped were never quite like my grand-mother's. Unattractive, lopsided, too loose, gooey preserves seeping from every crack imaginable—a far cry from the fabu-lous pastry cookies my grandmother's hands created. But she reassured me that I'd "have it down in no time." Whenever I think back on this memory today, I'm reminded to not only recognize but show appreciation for the special people in life who still cheer us on even when our performance or presenta-tion is nowhere near perfect. For me, Grandma was always my greatest cheerleader.

Cleanup was another special aspect of kitchen time. Dur-ing cleanup, when we noticed a raisin, chocolate chip, or rogue walnut nub lingering on the table, my grandmother and I wasted no time in treating ourselves to it. Like any good Italian with a healthy appetite, I now have a brain forever ingrained with the rule that food is never wasted, especially food items that are the occasional outlier from the weekly grocery budget, like chocolate.

In my grandparents' home, chocolate was a luxury.

Grandma and Bogey (a nickname my brother and I gave my grandfather) never were shy or embarrassed about their humble beginnings. This moment in life, the early 1980s, was simple—no Instagram highlight reels, no foodie posts. They were genuinely happy with the simple life they worked so hard to build. Grandma cooked or baked not for accolades but for the satisfaction she received when the family sat together eating in quiet contentment (a rare silence for us). As the food on our plates would begin to clear, a roar of laughter would erupt, followed by stories, news, updates about our lives, and reflection on the day's events. Most importantly, encouragement and love were generously apportioned among those at the table.

For some, those intimate human connections are missed in a busy world. For others, the dinner table is still a unifier; a daily act that requires so little of us yet provides an abundance of benefits. Eating together, research shows, means that members of a family exhibit better performance in work and school and children have closer relationships with parents and fewer issues

Fabulous Finds

The Perfect Indulgence

Chocolate is the perfect temporary indulgence—if your diet allows for it. And dark chocolate not only tastes amazing but is known for its mood-enhancing qualities due to its ability to raise serotonin levels. Aim for 70 percent cacao or higher to reap the most benefits.

with experimentation or later dependence on drugs and alcohol. Those who gather intentionally around the table also tend to make healthier food choices, including often subbing fruits and vegetables for fried, fatty foods and soda, in addition to gaining a more realistic view on food portion size. And repeated studies show that these regular gatherings help minimize the disconnection we can often feel due to busy work and school schedules, because they reconnect us with one another through sharing and storytelling and invite us to be present in the moment.[1] For my family, mealtime was a sacred act, and there was no excuse on God's green earth that would exempt you from missing it. In fact, if friends or other family members happened to be at the home during mealtime, guess what? They were eating too. End of story.

Now as an adult, childhood friends have shared with me that my grandmother's food and the act of eating at the table with my family remain one of the most poignant memories they hold. For me, that gathering around the table (and the kitchen time preparing) serves as a reminder that God created us for human connections—connections that reach beyond a ringing cell phone, chiming email, or technological distraction.

From early stories of scripture, Abraham showed hospitality to angel strangers. And the last supper Jesus shared was around a table, with both friends and an enemy. There was always a chair.

Even a short shared meal of thirty minutes can be beneficial, life-changing. (Though don't tell my family—they still believe some dinnertime events are meant to last an hour or more, depending on the occasion.)

From the customs my grandparents' generation held to the customs of Italian culture, large and lengthy mealtimes were our norm. Meals were meant to be shared and created community filled with family, friends, and neighbors. As children of

Italian immigrants, my grandparents grew up in New York with hopes of more suitable opportunities. Growing up, I watched a delicate balancing act take place in their home. While mealtime was a place of abundance, an economic recession mindset still resonated in other areas, ensuring indulgence or extravagance would not become commonplace in their home.

As I grew up, surrounded by life-giving forces and community, life almost seemed to be a revolving door of responsibilities that would teach me about frugality, including ripping napkins in half to double the amount before placing them on the table. Or reusing every glass jar you can get your hands on as a drinking glass or storage container, only turning on the air-conditioner once or twice a year, rolling pennies, hanging your wet clothes on the line (even if there was a clothes dryer), and saving the leftover lard after cooking.

The lard seriously disturbed me.

Each time I opened my grandparents' refrigerator for juice or a piece of cheese, swirls of brown and yellow fat, with an occasional crumb of food, stared back at me from a used glass jar that formerly housed olives. As I've grown, I've realized the magical content of this jar has transformative powers and adds delectable flavor to just about any dish that no amount of spice or culinary education could match.

Even with this realization, I've told no one. I've passionately protested against the lard jar for far too long, but even as a health and nutrition advocate, secretly I'm a convert to the taste. There is no going back.

Today I have my very own lard jar—a former home of pepperoncini; Grandma would be proud.

After our Saturday baking session, my grandmother and I would make our way outdoors while the rugelach cooled on a wire rack. Leisure was restorative. In my grandmother's eyes, that meant a cup of espresso, a good book, a cigarette, and a small square of rich, dark chocolate. We relaxed on the porch in wrought-iron chairs.

For anyone struggling with chronic illness or food issues and thinking, *Hmm, lard, espresso, cigarettes?* stay with me a minute. Hold a healing memory. We all have them, and we all will need them way into the future. And *your* healing moments might look very different. Hope and goodness and healing ways don't always look the same for everyone.

While my own health conditions and personal preferences don't allow me to partake in things like espresso or the occasional cigarette, I still hold these memories about my grandmother so dear to my heart. It was in these moments that I learned about self-care; I learned it was important to allow your body to rest after exertion; I learned we all should have a healing space where we can find solitude and peace, a place where we can collect our thoughts (for Grandma, this was definitely the porch); and that healing and joy can be found in the simple act of treating yourself to something you love. For my grandmother, it was espresso and chocolate; for me now it is usually a golden milk or chai tea and fresh fruit. And I am sure you have your own special treat that brings you a few moments of joy.

As we'd sit side by side, a warm, humid breeze dancing through the strands of our hair, I'd watch as my grandmother slowly unwrapped our dessert. Her thin fingers displayed a slight tremble, and I would study the deep lines etched into her always-smiling face. To some she may have come across as elderly, fragile, but in her I saw a fiery, free spirit living in an aging body, a person with a wealth of life knowledge, food knowledge, resilience knowledge. In later days she would teach me not only about cooking and the importance of community but also about not being defeated during rough seasons—as well as what it meant to be grateful for what God has given you, in plenty and in little.

Her presence in my life was one of my first glimpses of Jesus—of that spirit of kindness, compassion, and selflessness. She was also the person who taught me about the sacred, small healing act of sharing a precious piece of chocolate. And her commitment to preparing meals and assembling us around the dinner table would also be one of my first experiences of community. I learned we were somehow better figuring out life together than being separate.

As we sank deeper into the chairs, she would take a sip of the espresso and snap off a tiny piece of chocolate for me. I now treasure those moments of relishing in all we had just accomplished, nibbling on chocolate, content, not uttering a single word.

Chocolate Orange Rugelach

Prep Time: 40–45 minutes
Cook Time: 16–22 minutes, depending on your oven
Method: Oven
Yield: 48 rugelach

Even though I enjoy cooking, my love for baking is unmatched. Rugelach are my favorite desserts, in part because they remind me of time spent with my grandmother (in addition to tasting amazing). One of the best parts about any rugelach recipe is that you can get creative with it. I created this recipe with orange and chocolate—one of my favorite combinations—but you might want to swap out the orange for raspberry or add raisins and walnuts. Whatever you choose, they will likely come out delicious, and I bet you can't have *just* one!

INGREDIENTS

Dough
8 ounces of cream cheese, room temperature
½ pound unsalted butter, room temperature
¼ cup granulated sugar
¼ teaspoon salt
2 teaspoons vanilla extract
2 cups all-purpose flour (regular or gluten-free)

Filling
1 jar orange marmalade
One 14-ounce bar of bittersweet chocolate, crumbled or cut into
    tiny shavings and very small pieces
½ cup brown sugar
Cinnamon

Other Items
Parchment paper
Eggwash (1 egg beaten with 1 tablespoon milk or milk alternative)
Extra cinnamon and sugar for topping

In a stand electric mixer, cream your butter and cream cheese using a paddle attachment (if you prefer, cut butter and cream cheese into chunks before adding to your mixer). Pour in the sugar, salt, and vanilla and mix to combine. Keeping the mixer on low, add in the flour and mix just until combined. Do not overmix the dough or it will be tough.

Take the dough out of the bowl and place it on a floured surface. Shape it into a large ball (again, not overworking the dough). Separate the ball into four equal sections. Gently form each quarter into a ball shape, wrap in plastic wrap (not too tight), and put in the refrigerator for 1–1½ hours.

Cut or crumble your bittersweet chocolate (you want the pieces and shavings to be very small). Get your sugar, marmalade, and cinnamon ready. When the dough is ready to come out of the refrigerator, roll out each quarter into a 9-inch circle. You will have four 9-inch circles. Take 2 to 3 heaping tablespoons of marmalade for each circle. Spread the marmalade around each circle, getting all the way to the edges. Sprinkle the ½ cup sugar among all four circles evenly. Take your cinnamon spice bottle and sprinkle a light layer of cinnamon over each circle. Last, sprinkle your chocolate shavings/pieces over the four circles.

Now cut each circle into four quarters, and then each quarter into thirds. You should get 12 pieces of rugelach from each circle. Beginning with the wide edge, roll up each wedge. Place on a cookie sheet that has been lined with parchment paper, and lightly shape into a crescent. Chill the uncooked rugelach in your refrigerator for 30 minutes.

Take your rugelach out of your refrigerator once chilled and preheat your oven to 350°F. Lightly brush all rugelach with egg-wash and sprinkle a little extra cinnamon and sugar on top. Bake for 18–24 minutes (depending on your oven), until the top side is golden brown. Allow to cool before eating. Enjoy!

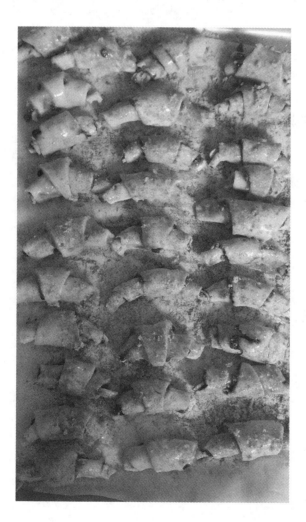

THREE

Seeing Potential—Even in the Fight of Your Life

God is more interested in your character than your comfort. God is more interested in making your life holy than . . . making your life happy.
—Rick Warren (adapted)

In the kitchen—appliances whirring, knives chopping, oil sizzling—my grandmother and I had a lot of laughter-laced discussions. Sometimes a more serious narrative would be woven into the threads of a larger tapestry of her life. Her storytelling itself was a multicolored cloth, a beautiful tapestry that was uniquely her own story.

Being able to afford meat regularly was out of range for us, and it wasn't uncommon to extend the life of a meat dish via numerous leftovers throughout the week. Just as her family had done when she was younger, everything was purposed and repurposed: a pot roast Grandma made on Sunday was stew by Tuesday and (my grandfather's favorite) hash as the week went on. "Be thankful for the food you are blessed with, Marisa," my grandmother always reminded me. "Always find a way to use your scraps in life—the things many will disregard as worthless have great value. And always," she added, "be grateful for a hot meal."

Her words linger with me. Living in a world where it can be easy to become swept up in the desire to have more, want more, or compare yourself to people who do in fact have more can sometimes lead us to be deficient when it comes to gratitude. This can also be said when it comes to chronic illness. It's no secret that a short time scrolling on social media can play tricks on your mind and might leave you feeling like someone else has more or someone has it better—better health, a better job, a better relationship. When this happens to me (and it definitely happens to me!), my grandmother's one sentence—"the things many will disregard as worthless have great value"—comes flooding back. Her words remind me to pause and check in on the blessings we all have in our life right now—to call on the wisdom spoken to us in our past to help us see today's challenges more clearly: Did we wake up this morning? Is there a roof over our heads and love in our home? Are we hungry, or are there various food options to create a meal from what is in our pantry and refrigerator? Even though that simple sentence was spoken to me over thirty years ago in my grandmother's kitchen, it continues to speak forth as a life lesson.

For my grandmother, this way of thinking was undoubtedly shaped by living through the Great Depression, and the way it influenced her culinary decisions was still evident in her kitchen. And in that very lesson, I finally understood the rationale behind the infamous lard jar—what one might quickly toss in the trash as waste, another would use over and over again to enhance what they already had.

Not too long after the Great Depression and food waste conversation, my ill-contained enthusiasm brought me to an unexpected discussion and introduced me to a side of my grandmother I was unfamiliar with. One early morning I ran to my grandmother's room, overeager to make homemade apple pies. In my impatience, I failed to knock, and barging in unannounced, I found my grandmother sitting on the corner of her perfectly made bed, which was covered with a colorful chintz quilt. She wasn't wearing a shirt and was tucking a small, oval-shaped pad into her bra. At that moment she looked frail and vulnerable, a stark contrast to the outspoken woman I spent time with in the kitchen. My body froze. We stared at one another, motionless, and the air suspended in my lungs until I caught my breath and, inquisitively, uttered the words, "Grandma, what's wrong with you?"

My initial smile melted into confusion as I saw the lightly raised, off-color scar stretching from her right armpit almost to the center of her chest. Any excitement about baking pies was turned into concern that something was seriously wrong with my grandmother. "It's okay. I am okay," she offered in a soothing voice. "Come sit . . ." Her left hand gently rubbed the quilt in a circular motion, summoning me. An overwhelming desire to wrap my arms around my grandmother poured over my body, and I raced to her. Even with so many questions, something told me to be in the moment and just be silent.

A short time later, pie dough was rolled out atop the floured glass kitchen table, and it was in this moment I learned about her breast cancer diagnosis, subsequent mastectomy, and fight for her life.

As it is for many of us, those rare and precious and meaningful moments are those we treasure and hold with us as healing memories. These are the moments we automatically go back to again and again. And so many pieces of this conversation would come back to me after I was struck by a vehicle and laid up in recovery, contemplating what my future held. Sometimes, my grandmother told me, we will go through a life season completely out of our control. Those seasons aren't a punishment from God or something we caused or something that is our fault. Cancer, she said, was this season for her.

And it was this baking session for me that introduced me to the lesson that life can suddenly swing in an unexpected direction. In that kitchen that day, I learned that fear for survival crossed her mind. And because survival is paramount when this season hits, if she wanted to continue doing the things she cherished and live out her life's purpose, she had to make a hard decision to put down some of her daily rituals and to-dos in order to take care of her body.

I could hear the urgency in her voice when she spoke about the cancer. She likened the experience to stepping into battle, and she taught me that you can only carry the things you absolutely need into battle in order to fight at the top of your game.

For her, stepping into battle called first for faith, and then food steps would be her secondary defense. In the brokenness and anxiousness she sometimes felt during this battle, food and faith fed her body in different ways each day. When her morale was low, she reached her hands out to her Creator. And when she felt physically weak, she consumed healing foods and herbs that would nourish her feeble body. "I didn't mind not sewing," she laughed. "And I could let go of the cleaning and the laundry . . . for a while. But cooking? Never. Cancer wouldn't be taking that." She smiled at me. "God always supplied me with the energy to cook."

As she shared the wisdom of her approach and told me stories of the pivotal life circumstances she faced, she spoke

Fabulous Finds

What You Always Keep

Remind yourself what chronic illness *cannot* take away from you:

Your hope

Your sense of humor

Your purpose

Your unique talents

Your beliefs

Your joy

Your kindness

Your ability to love

Your spirituality

Your rights

clearly, very matter of fact. In those years and later, she never pretended she was fully content when these hard seasons hit.

Another message I received from her in these conversations was that even in the midst of the life changes I would undoubtedly experience, they should not take away my kindness, my hope, my curiosity, my joy, and most importantly, my faith. She taught me to recognize that in many cases, a pivotal circumstance or uncomfortable season of change will do more for our character development and spiritual growth than any season of contentedness or blessing or bounty.

At the time, I didn't truly understand the value of the lessons I was given through these cancer conversations, but as I matured and reflected on my grandmother's struggle and the attitude she took to meet one of her most challenging seasons of her life, that attitude became a life preserver of sorts to me as I battled for my own life.

When we take time to recall those important conversations or return to a message we've been given from someone whose resolve has been tested, those glimpses of their response that we witness, their attitude toward the challenge in front of them, and how hard they were willing to fight are gifts from the struggle that they also are sharing with us. When my grandmother would share her stories, I imagined her a warrior, stepping into battle, covered in armor, sword in hand, unbeatable. In those moments, she wasn't the tiny, hundred-pound woman before me but this larger-than-life force to be reckoned with, the warrior who had already determined that defeat was unacceptable.

As I battled through my own tough season, I continued to draw hope, strength, courage, and a warrior-like determination from her. Not only were those lessons from her a compass of sorts, but I learned later that scientific studies confirmed what I knew about holding dear those lessons we've learned from our mentors.

Studies show that recalling autobiographical memories we associate with positivity can promote better well-being and is correlated with individual measures of resiliency. In addition, the capacity to savor the positive feelings we associate with that experience or memory corresponds to "an increased ability for emotional regulation, which in turn promotes successful adaptation to stress."[1]

So when it comes time to step into our own battles, we can know that those in our life who have stared death and illness and despair and strife directly in the face are on our team. We can join them to say to the challenge in front of us, "Not today! You lose; I will be victorious."

By the time we reach adulthood, we're well aware there is one constant in life—change. And most of us have a love-hate relationship with change at times. During difficult, stressful stretches, I try to remind myself of my grandmother's advice to not let these "growth spurts" diminish my joy or faith but rather let them deepen my faith, strengthen my resolve and trust in God's presence and care and greater wisdom in the situation. But change can be uncomfortable or scary, and we often respond with either fear or an attempt to avoid that change at all costs. There are seasons of life when things seem to go smoothly, full of repeated rhythms and patterns. And then in an instant, life happens. Some life changes come with happiness and delight—a wedding, the birth of a child, or hearing the words "You're in remission"—but there are other changes that don't give us joy or warm fuzzies.

In fact, when life radically shifts—and our momentary short-sighted perspective sees this change as a negative—we sometimes greet this unexpected (and possibly traumatic) development with a series of *Why* or *How* questions. And . . . in our anger and frustration, the first one getting the blast of our questions is usually God. We may have never even spoken to or thought about God before, but when a job loss occurs, a spouse requests a divorce, a loved one passes away, a pandemic hits, or a doctor tells us we have an incurable diagnosis, the floodgates open. We suddenly find ourselves at the intersection of ourselves, life events, and God, asking, *Why did this happen, God? How can you allow me to suffer like this, God?*

When I was recovering in the hospital, I had a long list of *Why* questions. Maybe they were immature, naive, but they were true questions. The questions came as heated accusations to God.

Why did you let this happen to me?

Are you there, God?

Hasn't life been difficult enough?

And in the bigger scheme of things, so many who are suffering ask, *Why do bad things happen to good people?*

I rescue dogs, I volunteer at nursing homes, I studied nursing to help other people, I take care of the elderly. If I'm a *good* person, then only good things should happen to me, *right*?

In the beginning stages of my recovery—call it weak faith or an inability to see a larger frame for the situation—my mind was desperately trying to find concrete answers as to why my current circumstance occurred.

The busyness of the hospital during the day—physician visits, blood draws, vital checks, and meals—reined in the emotional anguish for the most part. But things got ugly once the sun went down. When my slice of the world finally tucked itself in for slumber, my mind decided it was time to analyze every misstep, decision, trauma, or random life scenario . . . to death. The loneliness of the nighttime hospital setting only drove the pain into overdrive.

To quiet my thoughts, I'd tightly close my eyes and think back to kitchen days with my grandmother. Thankfully, these recollections remained vivid—ingredients, the viscosity of batter, the feel of the light from the window, the sound of her voice mixing with grit and resilience, offering up life lessons—and provided a safe space for my mind to finally achieve rest. The vast bank of memories my brain stored over the years served as the perfect distraction, even if only to get me through the long hospital nights.

With eyes closed, I could pretend I was no longer a prisoner in the hospital bed but instead at ease and propped up on a cherry-wood chair my grandfather had crafted for me in his garage workshop. He'd made it for me when I was tiny, giving me the exact boost needed to reach the kitchen countertop, allowing me to mash potatoes or evenly grease casserole dishes.

In the imagined chair, I can hear my grandmother's voice. I can even hear myself giggling as my tiny hands feed a slippery, slimy boiled potato into my grandmother's antique potato masher that looked like it was crafted when Jesus himself walked the earth.

Lying there, I was in another space, following instructions from my grandmother. She gave me a clearly defined task that would hopefully result in her famous garlic mashed potatoes. In my mind, I felt that excitement of complying, doing, creating.

My entire life I have been drawn to order, whether engulfed in a math equation or trying a new recipe. Because a recipe is methodical, reliable, and predictable, I find pleasure in knowing that a specific portion of this ingredient added to a precise portion of that ingredient renders the exact desired result time and time again. In these flashbacks, I find consistency and order and feel I am in control of my surroundings. Until a sudden cough, sharp pain, or IV alarm rips me back into reality, immediately reminding me of the present chaos that begs the question, *God, how did I wind up here?*

I wrack my brain for answers. Is this some kind of punishment? Did I do something wrong in my past? As humans, we search for answers. We are meaning seekers—trying to make sense of events or situations or decisions in life. We express a desire for closure, a longing for answers that will help us make decisions about a situation and a yearning to understand the *Whys* in life. Our inherent need to come up with answers (even if they aren't rational) when we are enmeshed in a cloud of uncertainty is an intrinsic part of our being human. The quest is as old as humanity. We see it time and time again—from the biblical narrative, to legends, to stories in pop culture, to our own search for answers in fields like psychology.

Social psychologist and distinguished University of Maryland professor Arie Kruglanski even coined the term *cognitive closure* back in 1989 to describe this behavior.[2] When, as humans, we need to eliminate ambiguity and obtain a straight answer, we try to bring cognitive closure. Each of us operates at a different level when it comes to our need for cognitive closure—or as we might say, a "need for closure," or NFC. Some of us lean toward a high NFC and prefer order, organization, and predictability, while others can tolerate indecision and open-ended situations, operating at a lower NFC.

Interestingly, our NFC increases if we are under pressure or fatigued, or have a lot of external distraction or noise directed toward us. Our NFC is also intimately tied to stress and peaks during times of crisis or in an emergency.

In my hospital bed, I found myself floating in a sea of questions, tracing the events that led to my hospital stay to future outcomes regarding regaining my health and independence. These questions, however, were impossible to answer in the moment. My need for closure was through the roof, but the well of answers was coming up dry.

At the very beginning of the hospital stay, my fragile body was exhausted and under the influence of too much medication to hold any type of meaningful or coherent conversation about the questions swirling in my head. But as days passed, I became more tolerant of the morphine drip and slowly regained my strength. One night, during a momentary burst of energy, I unleashed my questions to my mother, hopeful she could help me rationalize them.

My chin began to quiver and my eyes welled with tears as I tried to find the words: "Mom, d-di-id I do something to God? And now this is my punishment? Everything is gone. I have nothing left. I can't even walk."

She listened patiently as I cried out grievances—worry, and bitterness, and confusion. My immediate need to solve all problems lingered in the room between us, robbing the situation of any peace. Without judgment or pacifying platitudes like "Everything will be okay," instead she said, "Marisa, I don't have the answers for you, but I know a place you may find some clarity." While my grandmother could always be counted on for practical stories and life applications, my mother could be relied on to back every life circumstance with scripture and solid biblical knowledge. Leaning over her chair, she pulled out a tote to retrieve a small, tattered Bible. In my younger years, I didn't always have the patience for the stories and the antiquated language, but in the moment, I was hungry for answers and yearning to be fed.

"Why don't we look at Job?" she offered. Up to that point, my experiences in church were short Sunday masses at St. Bernard's Catholic Church around the corner from my grandmother's home, and I had the routine down—stand up, kneel, make the sign of the cross. What I didn't have was something deeper.

"Wait," I interrupted. "Does this story end with Job getting hurt and almost dying? This better be comparable to the crapshow I'm in. Because I need to hear about someone that would *really understand* what I am going through, Mom—and I'm looking for some hope too."

"Job understands what a difficult season is, *Marisa*," she responded. I noticed the usage of my full name, her Brooklyn-Italian accent descending in pitch and deviating in tone, signaling to me it was time to shut up and pay attention.

It turns out, the story of Job became the first story in the Bible I could relate to. The more I learned about this person who lost almost everything, the closer to God I began to feel. The more alive that tattered book was to me.

Job, considered one of the biblical books of wisdom literature, is one of the most painful yet beautiful stories in scripture.

It's full of descriptive prose, Hebrew poetry, rich characters, conversations, and declarations from God that reveal the magnitude of God's wisdom. And it takes on the big questions we all ask, like *Why do bad things happen?* and *Why do people suffer?*

The short version of the story is this: Job is a good man living in the land of Uz. He has a large family, land, cattle. God calls him righteous, a man "without blame." But a statement is made to God from the enemy that if everything was taken away from Job, surely he would curse God.

What follows is the loss of everything in Job's life—the only thing he doesn't lose is in fact his own life. His seven sons, his three daughters, his animals and caretakers, his home in a natural disaster—all gone.

As I listened to the story that he literally was left with only the clothes on his back, my mother read more about how at that point, he knew he had a choice. He tore the clothes from his body, fell to the ground, and got before God in a prayer that held pain and gratitude, loss and humility.

Mesmerized by Job's reaction and listening from the hospital bed about such devastation, I knew that when the first pang of pain hit me, I had approached God in anger. I had demanded answers. I realized that I never thanked, never listened. I just demanded. How could someone still be faithful when everything was broken? My brain attempted to understand this.

"It gets worse . . . ," my mother said, pulling me back into the story.

Another set of losses. This time the one thing Job has left is attacked—his health. Surely if he loses everything around him, his entire family, *and* his health, then he'll curse God. But Job responds again, unexpectedly, saying that as humans receiving unmerited blessings from God—our lives, families, homes—should we then turn from God the moment suffering comes upon us?

It's part of a much longer story of losses, faithless friends, and the difficult question about human suffering: When everything is lost, why does he not *curse God*?

Much of the remainder of this book is a long poetic discourse between him and his friends, who blame him and say that something he did must have brought on all this suffering. They say that if God is just and the universe runs on principles of justice, then that's the only explanation for why Job has lost everything. He brought it on himself. He did something wrong.

Finally, instead of focusing on blame and "what ifs" with his friends, Job demands that God show up in person and explain himself. And boy does God show up. In the form of a colossal whirlwind, God enters the conversation. But God never gives a specific answer to the question. In fact, he never even addresses it in the book.

Instead, God lays into Job and questions *him* about the complexities and expanse of the earth. God gives Job a tour of sorts of the cosmos where God outlines how expansive the world is, from its creatures to its most remote places, from the earth's measurements to the processes and functions of the entire universe.

God asks Job if he knows how to command the sunrise. And then God speaks to Job about the grace and freedom to be found in this wild and beautiful world. Job's viewpoint of the world is shattered yet expanded in this interaction with God. Job recognizes his limited perspective on life in light of the One who commands the laws of the universe.

And then something interesting happens before the book ends.

Looking back to that moment of my listening to the long story of Job, it was the first time I realized that instead of talking at, questioning, and accusing God, there might be a different way. What I learned from Job led me into my first-ever heart-to-heart with God.

As I listened to the story, things came into place. God told Job that the advice and explanations Job's friends gave him about God's justice and wisdom and why there was suffering in the world were all incorrect. And God told Job that his wrestling with the questions on his heart, his struggle in finding an answer, his honesty with God, and his conflict through prayer were good. In what follows, God tells Job to pray for his friends, and then Job is blessed with twice as much as the losses he suffered.

No simple or concrete answer to why bad things happen in our world. Only a limited human perspective. We may never know.

My grandmother never knew why she was diagnosed with cancer. I will never know why I was standing in the exact place I was when I was struck down by a truck. But in that hospital room, I knew I could bring the pain, questions, struggles, open heart, darkest seasons, and questions to God, a God I knew was with me in my brokenness and pain.

I don't believe it's a coincidence my mom told me the story of Job early on. I was at a pivotal point in my life. I needed to find someone I could relate to. In Job's story I saw that God could reach us through brokenness and suffering, to put a longing in our heart to reach out to Him when all else is lost. It was this story that shifted my perspective. For the first time, I felt I could put everything in my heart and mind out to God. It was life changing.

Job offered nuggets of wisdom for me, as someone reaching out to God. Job's prayers were true thoughts and raw feelings. And God listened. Job asked the Creator to speak. The prayers of Job continue to stay with me, reminding me to be honest, to wait, to listen, to be steadfast in prayer—even if times get more and more desperate (and they often do). And I learned, through Job's story and my own, that God responds—and the time frame and answers are not our own or about our demands, but they come from a deeper place of the God of the cosmos hearing the brokenness and listening.

After spending a few days on the story of Job with my mom sitting with me in the hospital room, she returned her frayed Bible to her purse and gathered her things to head home to be with my grandmother. "Can you turn off the lights on your way out, Mom?" I asked. And for the first time since I was admitted to the hospital, I was not dreading a night alone.

I was still held hostage by the hospital bed, forced to lay flat, to avoid putting pressure on my liver, but something had changed. In the quiet, I reflected on the possibility that faith and trust in God can exist in the middle of disaster.

After a long stretch of silence in the quiet, mostly dark room with a few flashing lights from my IV machines, an awkward whisper filled with hope released from my lips: "Hi, God. It's me, Marisa," I began.

Pizza Rustica / Easter Pie

Prep Time: 60 minutes
Cook Time: 70–75 minutes total
Method: Oven
Yield: 8 servings

My grandmother's pizza rustica recipe was probably the most treasured of all recipes in our home. This dish is hearty and delicious, though it does take some time to prepare. My grandmother often called it a "labor of love" that was well worth it, as she would smile wide while everyone in the house ate in silence, devouring this beloved dish. Though I can't personally eat it today with my specific health issues and allergies, it is my go-to meal when I have friends and family coming into town or when I want to make something special for the holidays.

INGREDIENTS

Dough
3½ cups all-purpose flour
1½ sticks unsalted butter, cold, cut into small cubes
¼ cup solid vegetable shortening, cold, cut into cubes (you can often find shortening in bars that resemble butter)
1 teaspoon Himalayan or sea salt
3 large eggs, beaten
3–4 tablespoons ice-cold water
One 9-inch springform pan

Filling
6 large eggs
One 15-ounce container of whole milk ricotta
One 8-ounce bag of shredded mozzarella
2 cloves garlic, pressed or minced
4 cups fresh baby spinach, coarsely chopped
4 ounces prosciutto, coarsely chopped   *(continued on next page)*

(ingredients continued)
¼ pound deli ham, coarsely chopped
¼ cup grated parmigiano reggiano cheese
4 ounces sliced pepperoni, coarsely chopped
¼ teaspoon salt
¼ teaspoon pepper
½ cup chopped fresh parsley
1 heaping teaspoon Italian seasoning

Topping
Eggwash (1 egg beaten with 1 tablespoon milk or milk alternative)

Begin by making your dough. Using a food processor, add your flour, cold butter, cold shortening, and salt. Blend together (toward the center of the food processor, it should look like a crumbly mixture). Add your eggs and pulse for a few seconds a few times in a row. Now as you pulse a few more times, you are going to slowly add your ice-cold water. Start with 2 tablespoons, then work your way up to 3 tablespoons (depending on the temperature and humidity level of your kitchen, you may only need 2 or 3 tablespoons of water). You'll know when you have added the right amount because a ball of dough will form quickly. Pulse a few more times so everything is combined, but do not overmix the dough. Place the slab of dough on a lightly floured cutting board and form into a large ball, again not kneading or overworking the dough. Now it is time to separate the dough into two balls of dough. I try to visualize the dough in thirds, making one ball about ⅔ of the dough and the other ball ⅓ of the dough. You will use the larger dough ball to line the bottom and sides of the springform pan and the smaller one to cover the filling. Once you have separated them, wrap them individually in plastic and place in the refrigerator for 30–45 minutes.

While the dough is in the refrigerator, it is time to make the filling for your pizza rustica. In a large bowl, combine your eggs, ricotta, mozzarella, garlic, baby spinach, prosciutto, ham, parmigiano reggiano, pepperoni, salt, pepper, parsley and Italian seasoning. Mix well until everything is combined. Set aside while you complete the next steps.

Generously grease your springform pan and preheat your oven to 375°F. On a floured surface, roll out the larger ball of dough into a 17/18-inch round. Line the bottom and sides of the pan and leave any extra dough hanging over the sides alone. Fill the springform pan with your wet mixture. Next, roll out the smaller ball of dough into an 11/12-inch round piece and drape over the filling. Now you can trim your dough, leaving enough excess from the top and bottom pieces to press them firmly into one another so the filling doesn't seep out. I press my dough into one another and then create a decorative edge with my fingers or using a fork. Brush the top of the pie with some of your eggwash. Also, poke a few holes in the top of the pie to let steam through while cooking.

The pizza rustica needs to be placed on the bottom or second to bottom rack (I put mine on the second to bottom rack) and cook at 375°F for 70–75 minutes, or until a fork placed in the center comes out clean. Remove from oven and let sit for 20 minutes or so before removing from springform pan and serving. Enjoy—this is going to be delicious!

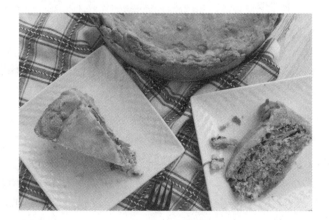

FOUR

A Lesson in Silence

There is purpose in your season of waiting.
                                        —Megan Smalley

According to my mother, I've always been a talker. In fact, she still tells stories of me "waking up with the birds" as a baby either singing or having incoherent conversations with myself. Whether in song or spoken or written word, I've always had something to say.

Despite my love for communication, the truth is, my first few prayers with God after I heard the story of Job rambled and drifted and were incredibly awkward. I second-guessed myself. *Am I supposed to be praying a certain way?* I second-guessed God. *Is God listening? Is this all too trivial for God?*

It's a struggle most of us face when we are at the point in our life we feel we must reconsider our understanding of our faith, our belief in a higher power, our relationship with a supreme being. With all that is going on with us, and with all that is going on in the world, we might wonder, Do our prayers even matter? Will they even be heard?

For me, God—that supreme being—was one I needed to reconcile with. With wars, and famine, and human trafficking, and cancer, and violence, and racism, and all plights that countless people across the earth face, I had to ask, Do we matter to God? And how much weight do my words have in the eyes of God? And do I matter?

I wondered if I should keep going. I hesitated—a lot. But when I stopped, it was like a barrier came up. And I thought about Job, on his knees, clothes torn, talking it out with the Almighty: letting loose, true feelings, all of it. I told myself the awkwardness wouldn't last forever, and the first few times anyone tries anything it is usually a hot mess. Like that disastrous time I tried snorkeling lessons. So I talked and practiced, I prayed and voiced all of the questions out loud, and then the dam metaphorically broke. Right there from my hospital bed. And my words to God haven't stopped gushing since.

Any relationship requires ongoing communication. It isn't always comfortable in the beginning, but over time a fulfilling and deep relationship begins to form between you and that person, built on honesty, trust, and deep dialogue. Over time you realize, when the onrush of talking settles, that something else emerges, silence. Listening. And that brings the relationship to an even deeper level.

Silence allows us to listen and hear each other, to learn and absorb information, and to reflect or take pleasure in a moment. Perhaps one of the most beautiful examples of a silence that is generative and one that you have likely experienced is when you are with a good friend or a beloved partner and you mutually delight in the stillness and quiet, not having to utter a single word.

In silence, we can also calm our physical bodies *and* our souls. For many of us, when we find our bodies aren't working the way we hoped—when we meet a health crisis or when we're no longer able to function the way we once did—there's a kind of noise and panic that comes out. And the more noise we meet, accept, or create, the less we can listen and understand. And when we meet the limits of our bodies, the soul place can offer us wisdom. And the soul place doesn't have the limits of the body space. But silence doesn't necessarily come naturally for most of us, especially when we are smack-dab in the middle of a trial or challenging season.

In the spiritual realm, silence brings us an opportunity to not only hear God but also sense God's presence. In Hebrew scripture, there's a story of the prophet Elijah, whose life is threatened, and he runs to the wilderness. In the silence, he finds the courage he needs. And Job, trying to reconcile his season of suffering, sits in silence with his friends for seven days.

Our bodies want to *do things*—achieve, move, act. And our minds can get so busy that they don't stop. We make noise, mulling it over and over, as though not stopping and just doing and thinking, we will have more control over the situation. But what I learned after the talking and in the silence was listening. Stopping allowed me to be still and listen to a voice that wasn't just my own, to gain wisdom about the situation.

Anyone who has meditated, learned to pay attention to the breath, or prayed, knows that there are not only spiritual benefits from the silence but also physiological and psychological advantages. The human body actually thrives on peace and stillness. In fact, silence is known to boost the immune system and promotes good hormone regulation. It also benefits our brain. A 2013 study in *Brain Structure and Function* found that silence can actually help brains grow new cells; more specifically, two hours of silence regenerated new cells in the hippocampus area of the brain in mice, an area associated with memory, learning, and feelings and reactions.[1] Another study in *Heart*, this one focusing on humans, revealed that just two minutes of silence was more beneficial to the brain than listening to two minutes of relaxing music—not only did the silence decrease one's heart rate, but it also improved blood pressure readings and increased blood flow to the brain.[2]

Physiologically and psychologically, silence and stillness allow you time for true reflection and can prove quite helpful—especially when you are experiencing a challenging season. Without all of the external stimuli, you finally have an opportunity to tap into your feelings and ideas and better connect with and organize your thoughts and memories. When you find yourself in a state of silence, your default mode network in your brain, also known as DMN, is engaged.[3] Your DMN is a group of brain regions, and once it is engaged—by taking part in introspective activities such as meditating, daydreaming, letting your mind wander, and fantasizing—you dip below the surface layers of the mind and begin to play back, contemplate, and make meaning out of the experiences you have had. It offers the opportunity for you to consider the perspectives of other people, provides room for your creativity to blossom, and helps you begin to think about what your future may hold.

Once outside noise and influence are cut off, in the quiet moments, you also become more aware of yourself, your mental and emotional state, and your environment. It is a beginning place where you can recalibrate and heal. And every single part of your being benefits when you choose to rest in the silence and escape the noise.

Those first few days in the hospital, in the trauma intensive care unit (TICU), my barely coherent body—disrupted by

Fabulous Finds

Discovering Silence

Take advantage of the benefits of meditation and silence. Even just a few minutes a day can

- lower blood pressure
- lower cortisol levels
- boost the immune system
- allow for greater reflection
- increase creativity
- improve sleep quality

excruciating pain and then infused with painkillers—began to learn silence. As I became more tolerant of the sedating drugs though, I struggled to free myself from the noise. The "noise" for me was rooted in fear. My mind was constantly mulling over the events that had just taken place, the fear and lack of control and loss of independence. I kept verbally and mentally rehashing all I had remembered about the event with my mom, hoping I missed a clue somewhere that would make sense of everything. I wanted to keep talking to avoid the pause. That same pause that so many of us want to ignore or fight off. That pause where we aren't so overloaded and busy and we have to actually face, head-on, the challenges that are staring right at us and the heavy, uncomfortable feelings that are attached to them. Most of us are so used to living in a world with excess noise, we rarely sit in silence to ground our thoughts and let our body, mind, and soul actually begin to heal.

The TICU I was in was probably one of the quietest places in the hospital. Sounds strange, right? For those familiar with hospital settings, what often stands out is the barrage of beeps, dings, and alarms coming from medical devices that often disrupt the peace of a patient. Lights are often on at intense levels. Doors are open so that those from the circular nurse and physician station can view patients twenty-four hours a day.

But I noticed that this unit was different. The medical staff seemed on high alert to reduce the level of noise if it became unsettling. Here, they actually seemed to value the importance of silence and rest and its ability to restore a hurting body.

At first, at night, I began to fight the silence. All I wanted to do was sit up straight, get out of this bed, walk around, be in my own home, get back to college . . . not pee in a bedpan—the list was endless, really. But I could barely lift a leg or talk for more than a few minutes without being overwhelmed with exhaustion, so lying there, I was forced to learn the art and discipline of being *silent* and learning to *listen*. These two words go hand in hand with one another, and I don't think it is an accident that they are spelled with the same letters.

You can hear a lot when you have no choice but to listen. I could soon determine when a new visitor had arrived on our floor; when my IV bag was empty; when my heart was experiencing a calm, rhythmic beat; and when the second hand of the clock hanging on the wall to my right was making its way between the fifty-five- and sixty-second mark, as its sound increased. In listening, I learned about the gentleman in the room next to me, as physician and family conversations occurred in the hallway. While I was listening to the conversations, a nurse came in to check on the morphine drip and noticed I was paying attention to the hallway conversation. "You're one of the lucky ones," she told me, the only one on the floor right now who was conscious. What she said grabbed my attention. *Are the others listening too?* I wondered. *What can they hear in their current state?*

I began to fixate on the word *lucky*. I was the only one in the unit who could engage with others, who could listen to my mom as she read the story of Job from her tattered book. I was the only one able to communicate with medical staff when I needed to, and I was able to recognize the silence growing, as hospital personnel finished rounds and visitors were leaving for the day.

It's been said that silence is the beginning of listening. In the placid moments of nighttime, I felt I was given a set of choices. I could let my mind run wild, fueled by fear and frustration, or I could choose something different. I saw the opportunity to pray my heart out and to listen for God. And the more I chose to pray, the more I listened. And the more I sensed God. And then I began to see small, positive shifts in my outlook and my thinking patterns.

Yes, unfortunate circumstances led me there, but right at that moment, I had a quiet, still season to listen to God, with very little distraction happening around me. *Will I ever get another opportunity like this in my lifetime?* I wondered.

There was no neatly packaged answer for why the suffering occurred in the first place, no answer to the question I originally asked, but the situation slowly began to swing in more quiet, optimistic directions.

My questions shifted. Instead of wondering, *Why is God doing this?* I began to reflect, *What is God doing with me through this?* My brain shifted from its default negative-patterned programming of seeing the event only as one of suffering (which it was) to slowly teasing out the possibility that there could also be blessings somewhere in this circumstance. Perhaps that was the hardest shift in the thought process to make—to not see things as solely good or bad but rather to see a challenging or traumatic experience as something that may refine me in some way, build my character, show me how much stronger I actually am than I give myself credit for, or impress on me to pause every now and then and soak in the joy that is in my life.

I began to look at things differently. Slowly. *What if prayer and silence*, I wondered, *are the key for us to recalibrate so we can listen to what is around us and hear both the voice of God within and our own true voice?*

I lay in my hospital bed and studied the grain and texture of the ceiling tiles for the hundredth time, rubbing the thin, scratchy hospital blanket between my thumb and forefinger, and suddenly I recognized a feeling I hadn't felt in a long time— contentedness. In the middle of the pain running through my body and the recurring beat of the IV machine dispensing its life-sustaining medication, I sensed that something was changing, that something bigger than that moment of crisis or moment of pain was at work.

As I continued to have conversations with my mom about what I was learning about God and faith and silence, I didn't expect that our following conversations would again veer in a very different direction so soon.

. . . .

"The reward you get for overcoming your last challenge," Bishop T. D. Jakes once said, "is your next challenge."[4] As someone who was only beginning to understand what it meant to meet new challenges and how to navigate them, I thought, *Well, I went through a horrific experience, I survived it, and life will be nice and quiet now, right?*

A few weeks into my recovery, I woke up with a fever that lasted and lasted. The medical team thought the fever was likely caused by an infection, but they couldn't find any infection. Tubes of blood were drawn and tested over several days. No answers.

More blood was taken from the needle placed in my arm, the deep red liquid spiraling down skinny tubing into two small containers that reminded me of minibar vodka bottles. Three days later, the blood cultures showed nothing. Again, no infection.

Weeks into my time at the hospital, I hadn't moved. Every time I tried, I was completely exhausted. My doctors tried to discern if the exhaustion and body aches were the result of being hit by the truck or if they had a separate origin. As the fever raged, a pinkish-red rash appeared on the trunk of my body and across my face. My nose and mouth broke out in painful sores. The doctors kicked around the idea of a virus . . . until the left side of my face started going numb and the left side of my bottom lip began to droop one afternoon.

No budding faith kicked in.

No poster child showed up living into the mantra "If God brings you to it, God will bring you through it."

Nope. Nothing.

I wish I could tell you I reacted in a cool, calm, and collected manner to my newfound lip sag, but my reaction was quite the opposite. Feeling around for my compact in a small makeup bag I kept on the bed for easy access, I opened it to access the mirror and stare at my saggy lip, pushing it into its proper position over and over only to watch it wilt back down once again. *Something is wrong*, I said to myself. Soon, my heart started beating faster and harder. The vitals machine above my head sounded. And I clutched at my throat as classic symptoms of a panic attack suddenly drove through my body like a freight train. I repeatedly mashed the nurses' call button and yelled out, "Hello! I need help! Hello!?"

A variety of new tests, consults, and scans later, we finally got an answer: a ministroke. I didn't know then that this answer would lead to another set of answers about what was happening in my body. The team of physicians debated whether this ministroke was related to the head injury sustained when my skull crash landed into the asphalt, to my blood circulation, or to a potential clot from lying in bed for so long or had occurred because of an entirely different reason altogether.

My room became a revolving door for specialists from infectious disease and rheumatology. Terms I was unfamiliar with suddenly were constant: rheumatic fever, tick-borne diseases, HIV, rheumatoid arthritis, and tropical diseases with names I still can't pronounce. The physicians seemed confident that whatever was causing the myriad symptoms, they would find it. I actually felt optimistic, believing that if strange medical symptoms were to ever happen in my life, being overseen by a team of doctors in the hospital was probably the best situation for this to occur.

See what just happened there? It was during instances like this—that I reflect on today—that small shifts in my mindset started to occur. Yes, I was so utterly terrified and confused about what was happening to my body, but at the same time, I was so grateful that out of all the places in the world I could be, I found myself in a top hospital surrounded by incredible physicians. The blessing was peeking out and beginning to pour some light on all the darkness that seemed to be hovering around me.

Now, even though I had confidence in my medical team, I didn't have quite as much confidence in my body. Between my initial injuries from being hit and these new symptoms, my body suddenly seemed foreign to me. Within this body that stored everything that is *Marisa*, my thoughts and what was physically taking place were disconnected, seemingly different universes. The truth was, I had no control over my body, and it felt almost as though a betrayal were taking place, that every cell conspired to attack me as payback for all that transpired. Thinking back, my perception of the situation wasn't that far off.

"Marisa, have you ever heard of systemic lupus?" I stared at the rheumatologist's shiny jet-black hair that was perfectly styled into a French bob.

"Um, what? I have no idea what that is or what you even just said," I mumbled. We spoke for twenty minutes, but the only three things I remember are these:

1. I now have what is considered an autoimmune disease.

    Currently, the National Institutes of Health estimates almost twenty-four million people in the United States live with an autoimmune disease. I am now part of this tribe.[5]
2. There is no magic pill when it comes to curing auto-immune disease.

    In fact, there aren't many options or answers at all, especially when it comes to autoimmune disease. Currently, more than one hundred autoimmune diseases have been identified, and lupus is just one in that list—one that happens to be severely lacking in research and treatment options. And according to the American Autoimmune Related Diseases Association (AARDA), most people who are diagnosed with an autoimmune disease will wait an average of three years or more for a diagnosis, be referred to four to five doctors, and spend around $50,000 to discover why they are sick.[6] For me, even though I can clearly recall lupus symptoms from a young age that were consistently ignored, I received a speedy diagnosis by having all of the tests completed in the hospital and being seen by multiple teams of doctors all at once.
3. Sometimes, the symptoms of the disease are exposed after a trigger (physical trauma, severe illness, or even pregnancy). My trigger was the collision with the three-thousand-pound truck.

"So if I didn't get hit by the truck, I may not have gotten sick?" I asked the rheumatologist.

"I can't tell you these symptoms wouldn't have occurred at some other point in your life, but in this case the physical trauma on your body seems to be the catalyst," she informed me.

"Okay, so what can I do to get rid of it?" I responded, optimistically putting this statement out into the universe.

My optimism lasted about three seconds.

"There is no cure for lupus, but we can try some different medications to manage it," she replied.

No cure, more medicine? What if I didn't get hit by the truck? Those lines became a track that started playing on repeat in my head after the specialist left my room. This tiny five-letter word opened a chasm in the universe that I felt was about to swallow me whole. Suddenly, I realized I was ill prepared for whatever was coming next with this strange-sounding disease, unaware I was about to get a lifetime of education.

Noticing the spiral I was about to head down, I tried to focus on the stillness in the room, to bring peace to my mind. Then I closed my eyes and started talking to God. Surely if anything could help me calm the thought circus on the center stage of my mind and help me feel less like I was about to fall into an abyss, it would be prayer.

This sounds really bad, God! was how I started. *And I am really scared about what is happening to my body. Please teach me to see the blessing in this somehow through the fear and find some peace, because right now all I can focus on is my worry and anger and heartache.*

. . . .

My prayer eventually transformed into rest and one of the deepest sleeps I had had in a while, until it was abruptly broken by the exuberant and feisty spirit of my grandmother entering my hospital room with trays of food. "You no eat enough, Marisa! That's why you no feel good," she exclaimed loudly. "You skin and bones!" she added as she put down the food and lifted my limp wrist from my side. Seconds after her entrance, a gaggle of other family members seemed to descend on my room.

The minute Italian family members find out you are sick and in the hospital, they immediately do several things:

- Cook for you
- Feed you
- Feed you again
- Tell you at least a dozen times that you aren't eating enough or do not weigh enough and *this* is the sole reason you became sick.

Regular visits in the hospital from my cousin, aunts, uncles, mom, and grandmother brought food and lectures and broke the monotony, lifting my spirits. I secretly looked forward to the gourmet food they brought each day without fail (even if it came with unsolicited, bizarre advice and opinions about my health).

In stressful situations, I tend to lose my appetite, but each dish arrived, too mouthwatering to deny. Italians believe there is no illness enough garlic, lemon, onion, chicken broth, and brandy or amaretto won't heal. And with my newly added diagnosis, a battle of the kitchens emerged to see whose meal was going to make me magically feel better.

I welcomed their unstated but obvious competition; one more serving of bland hospital rice pilaf and prepackaged chocolate pudding would send me over the edge. And don't even get me started on the cans of oil-based chocolate shakes medical staff pushed on me, saying, "Calories, Marisa, calories." Um, gross, hospital personnel . . . just gross.

These lovingly prepared home-cooked meals became a topic of nightly conversation on the floor among the nurses and me as the savory aroma would lead them into my room. Would tonight's meal be stuffed peppers, sausage and potatoes with onions, or Grandma's famous pizza rustica? Whatever the culinary masterpiece, I was gifted with so much more than a supply of nutrition and energy to my body.

As the dinner table was brought to my hospital room each night, I began to reconnect not only to the outside world but also to myself. I was injured and now faced a disease as well, but I was conscious, I could eat on my own, and I was still able to enjoy one of my favorite daily activities—sharing a delicious meal with my family.

In brief, dinner-length moments, this daily custom helped me forget I was in recovery. As I devoured each dish, I quietly watched my family—those people God put into my life—interacting with one another. There were laughter, bits of food stolen off each other's plates, details on how the dish was prepared, and theories as to why each kitchen's way was, of course, the *only* way it should be made.

At dinnertime, we forgot the sadness that overcame our family when I first arrived at the hospital. Instead, we found joy and our smiles once again.

Mom would slide her arm between the bars of the hospital bed and give my right hand a long, gentle squeeze. Smiling, she would whisper, just loud enough for me to hear, "We aren't going to let this new situation, this test, harm our faith, Marisa. God knows exactly why all of this is happening and is going to use it for good. Maybe not tomorrow, or next year, but in the right time. Just you watch."

As she said this, my cousin walked over and placed a small bowl of homemade rice pudding on my lap. "Come on, bones, it's time for dessert." My favorite. The sweet cream and cinnamon flavor lightly wrapped around my tongue and was a welcome treat after a rich, salted meal. And instead of thinking about my bright-red rash, or relentless fever, or strange, sharp pains in this moment, I looked around and witnessed the blessing unfolding in front of me—the blessing that was right before my eyes, that I could have missed if I had failed to focus on what was in front of me.

This is my *family,* I thought. *And they are pretty fabulous.*

Nerves were quickly abated by hope. Worry shifted to look something like budding faith. I said to myself, *I may not know what my future holds, but I do know that right here, right now, I am safe. I am loved. And in the deepest recesses of my human understanding of the Creator, I am confident God is not going to let me down.*

It's sitting in that space, the one where you tell yourself you are loved and safe and capable of triumph, that helps you hold onto hope whatever the situation, whatever the news. It is deciding to dig deep to find the blessing—however small—amid the crisis or disaster, the one blessing that can help you from spiraling down into an abyss. And it is the decision to reflect in silence and engage in listening that allows you to receive the message that this hardship, this challenge will not be the very end of you but in fact may be the very thing that drives an insatiable desire to rejoice in living.

Stuffed Peppers

Prep Time: 25 minutes
Cook Time: 35–45 minutes total
Method: Saucepan and oven
Yield: 8 servings

Like many Italians, one of the shared meals I grew up on was stuffed peppers. Eating it together with my family, I think, *Not only is this meal fabulous, but these people at the table are fabulous.* One reason I love this recipe (besides the fact that it is delicious) is that the recipe is so versatile. You can sub ground chicken or turkey for the ground beef or even use a vegetarian meat substitute and it will still turn out incredibly tasty. Plus, you can add different herbs and spices according to your preference. Cook time is also something you can play with; I prefer to cook my peppers on the longer side until they are soft and can be easily pricked with a fork, but some people prefer their peppers with a bit more crunch and choose to cook them for less time. Also, I make this recipe with rice, but you can sub quinoa or another grain you have in the pantry.

INGREDIENTS

8 bell peppers, any color, washed and seeded
2 tablespoons olive oil
1 medium yellow onion, diced
1 pound ground beef
4 cloves garlic, pressed or minced
1 cup sliced white mushrooms
2 cups fresh baby spinach
½ cup fresh chopped basil, separated in half
1 cup cooked rice (white, brown, jasmine—your choice)
One 14.5-ounce can petite diced tomatoes
One 6-ounce can tomato paste

(continued on next page)

(ingredients continued)
¼ teaspoon salt
¼ teaspoon black pepper
1 package shredded mozzarella, separated in half

Preheat your oven to 350°F. Wash peppers, cutting tops off and removing all seeds from the inside. Place pepper tops off to the side. In a large pan, heat olive oil on medium heat. Sauté your onion until it becomes golden brown and then add your ground beef and garlic. Stir and cook until your meat is brown. Next, add your mushrooms and spinach and cook for a few minutes until both are cooked or wilted. Add half of the fresh chopped basil, cooked rice, diced tomatoes, tomato paste, salt, and pepper and stir well. Cook for a minute or so and turn off heat. Leaving pan on heat source, add in half of your shredded mozzarella cheese and stir to combine and melt.

Next, take a large casserole dish (I typically grease mine with more olive oil), fill peppers with mixture from saucepan, and place next to each other in the casserole dish. Sprinkle the remaining mozzarella cheese on top of the peppers. This next step is optional, but I like to cover my pepper with its lid before I place it in the oven to bake. Bake on middle rack for 35–45 minutes; the longer you cook it, the softer and more wilted the pepper will be. Top with fresh basil when cooked, serve while hot, and enjoy!

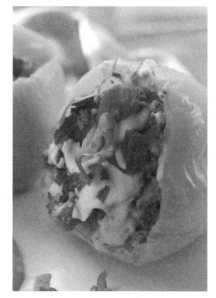

FIVE

Timelines and Triggers

*What if this painful breaking is part
of a beautiful remaking?*
—Lysa TerKeurst

*She stood in the storm and when the wind did
not blow her way, she adjusted her sails.*
—Elizabeth Edwards

Look closely enough, and you can often witness the turning point in any challenging situation—that moment a tiny sliver of hope creeps in and shines the faintest light in a sea of darkness. It's a shift that can occur when we are facing a challenging season with a spouse, grief over the loss of a loved one, or some other tragedy that knocks us temporarily from our foundation. My sliver came in the form of discharge papers from the hospital, leaving me to the care of my family full time, with trips to a rehabilitation center three days per week.

I sat on the edge of my bed, feet dangling, with an unfocused stare in the direction of the nurses' station. Though I had been looking forward to this moment for some time, a few unsettling thoughts crept in. My injuries improved each day, though I couldn't fully walk on my own. I was still on shaky ground when it came to the lupus. The medical staff had been helping me with medical details and care instructions, but soon it would all fall on me and my family. *How will I do this without them?* I wondered.

"All right, Marisa! Are you ready to break out of here!?" a bubbly hospital transporter exclaimed as she swung a black wheelchair into my room, breaking my concentration. My mother standing next to me, brief goodbyes were exchanged with hospital staff, along with awkward, side-bodied wheelchair hugs. As we inched closer to the elevator, I glanced at the other people on the floor, connected to tubes and machines keeping them alive. My mom looked at me with an attempted smile, but instead her eyes filled with tears. I half-smiled, half-cried back. Sadness, gratitude, and relief all were expressed in this brief, wordless exchange. We understood the difficulty of the journey ahead for those men and women still in battles; we met a gratitude, too, for surviving what many thought wasn't survivable and a relief that this chapter of this story would come to a close almost as swiftly as it began.

Arriving at home, my mom and grandmother helped me into a smaller, collapsible wheelchair and maneuvered me to my bedroom.

Everything was exactly as I had left it.

The comfort of returning to the solace of my room was met with a twinge of bitterness that welled up when I saw my belongings and my homework spread out across my desk, my work clothes in a pile near one corner.

It was as though I stepped into an alternate universe, one where life went on as usual in this room . . . just without me. But it didn't. And now I returned with the task of figuring out how to blend my current reality with one I didn't want to give up in the first place—a reality that no longer existed. I was still alive, but I was not the same Marisa who left her homework. This would in fact be the moment that changed my perspective forever—now putting everything into the categories of "Life before I Was Hit" and "Life after I Was Hit," "Life before I Got Sick" and "Life after I Got Sick." And everything in front of me in this bedroom was "Life Before" . . . and it felt like a cruel joke.

A torrent of emotions hit me, emotions I was completely unprepared for. You may have experienced something similar after a loss or sudden illness, whether it was a loss of a loved one and you've returned home to the place his or her personal belongings and cherished items still take up residence or you've lost your physical health or independence. There is really no way to plan for or prepare yourself for this type of event until you actually experience it. And when you do experience it for the first time, it almost feels like the ground under your feet disappears. In that moment, your mind wrestles and struggles, trying to figure out how to exist in two completely opposite realities—life before, life after. You feel lost in a new unknown.

For me, I was surrounded by items that seemed frozen in time from my former life as an independent college student, and somehow I was now supposed to work into my previous world a disabled body that had next to no independence. It was a puzzle piece from a separate box, and there was no possible way on earth a seamless fit was going to take place. These two worlds could never overlap, and something was not going to make it through this transition.

"I'd like to sleep for a while," I announced, avoiding eye contact with my mom, who helped me into the bed, and my grandmother, who stood at the door. I gave them every indication that I was tired, but I didn't sleep right away. Within the bitter was the sweet, and I savored this first moment of truly being alone in so very long. I turned my back to my room, away from the memories of the things I had missed so much, and faced the wall, tucking my face deep into the pillows, sobbing.

I wasn't even sure why I was crying. Perhaps it was the result of an overwhelming surge of emotions. Perhaps it was frustration and anger flowing out of me. Perhaps it was the only way I knew how to express to God *Thank you for not letting me die that night* alongside the anguished prayer *What in the world happens now?* I cried myself into hours of a deep sleep.

My return home consisted of sleeping, eating, having medical personnel come to assess my progress, and spending two or three times longer than usual to complete any simple activity of daily living, like bathing, which took up most of my day and energy.

"If opening your eyes, or getting out of bed, or holding a spoon, or combing your hair is the daunting Mount Everest you climb today, that is okay," writes author Carmen Ambrosio, who lives with multiple sclerosis.[1] Her words resonated with me.

When you are recovering from a physical injury or devastating health challenge, everyday actions can literally feel like you *are* climbing Mount Everest with no physical or emotional reserves to do so.

Once you need help to do the simplest tasks, you realize how much energy it took for it took to do things like washing yourself, brushing your teeth, making breakfast, or getting dressed. Most of us never give those activities much thought if we haven't been impacted by physical injury or illness. In fact, the tasks may have seemed almost robotic and might have been completed without too much thought involved. And then suddenly you are spun into a world where you have to almost create an FBI link diagram (or "crazy wall" as some call it) just to map out, connect, and make a plan of action regarding the main elements in your life related to feeding, bathing, and dressing yourself.

When not spending an hour attempting to put on pants and a T-shirt, or two hours getting undressed and into a bathtub, I spent time reconditioning my body. Three days per week, my mom dropped me off at a rehabilitation center where we worked on rebuilding lost muscle and strengthening my body in order to graduate me from wheelchair, to walker, to eventually walking on my own.

From beginning with exercises and weights while I was sitting in the wheelchair, to standing in front of the wheelchair, to—within a few weeks—graduating to a walker (tennis balls on the feet and all), the exertions were exhausting. Walking for one minute with the walker, my legs would shake violently. I would become so frustrated that a simple, short exercise would wipe me out for the rest of the day. The medical team recognized my need for encouragement, and they reminded me of how much I'd improved in just a short time frame.

My mom, on the other hand, would remind me not to get lost in the comparison trap of my life now versus my life a few months ago: "Look at how far you have come, Marisa. Change your perspective." The physical therapist reminded me again and again that I was battling not just the aftermath of a traumatic event and muscle atrophy from time in the hospital but also fatigue and pain from the lupus. He would speak life over me by continuously telling me—even though I didn't believe it at the time—"how resilient" I was.

I thought a lot about the term *resilience* during my long stretch in bed throughout recovery. Where I sometimes felt like a complete failure, someone barely able to get through a set of rehab exercises, other people viewed me with a sense of amazement, somewhat in disbelief that I had literally survived getting hit by a truck and a life-challenging diagnosis.

You may have experienced this as well, where you feel like you are barely holding it together during a crisis, but other people are looking to you as a source of inspiration—a role model. So what actually makes us resilient?

Resiliency is this ability to cope with a setback, to withstand and recover from a challenge. It's having a reservoir of strength that you can draw on when everything around you seems to be falling to pieces. When a disaster hits—like a diagnosis, a divorce, or the loss of a loved one—it doesn't mean the resilient person experiences less distress and pain and anxiety and sadness; it means they handle the situation in a different manner. Where one person might become distraught, overwhelmed, and completely focused on the problem, causing them to lean on negative coping mechanisms that can cause damage and destruction in their life, the resilient person digs deep into their arsenal of skills and strengths in order to make it through. The resilient person envisions themselves as a warrior rather than a victim of the situation, can effectively manage and regulate their emotions, typically has higher self-esteem and a positive image of themselves, and is motivated to take the actions necessary to survive the situation because they are led by an internal locus of control.[2]

Research professor and author Brené Brown is known for speaking about resilience. In her research and in her book *The Gifts of Imperfection*, she shares that in the person with the resilient spirit, we also tend to see a willingness to reach out to others for help, resourcefulness, problem-solving skills, and a rooted connection to friends and family. Brown also discovered that resilient people are often people who are spiritual—their spirituality isn't necessarily tied to one specific religion, but rather they sense a connection to a power greater than themselves, grounded in love and compassion.

And perhaps one of the best aspects of resiliency is that you don't have to be a naturally resilient person. You can actually build resiliency in yourself over time by focusing on the things you can control and not getting stuck in the mindset of wanting to go back in time to the "way things were before." You can build resiliency through a circle of supportive people you can trust and confide in, people you feel comfortable sharing your challenges with and having the hard and uncomfortable conversations with. Resiliency is also built when you look for small, positive ways to foster growth and tackle problems associated with your challenges—instead of getting stuck in a loop of negative emotions and thinking patterns. By handling life's challenges in this way, we make it possible for ourselves to grow and to emerge even stronger than we were before the disaster occurred.

Though I felt like I was fighting two demons at once—the injuries from being hit and now the illness—and I sometimes considered how much easier rehabilitation would have been if I were only trying to overcome injuries, I refused to give in. Instead, my brain wanted to solve the problems that lay before me. I had a lot of questions, and I was hungry for answers.

One day after rehab, I lay in bed and thought back to the conversation with the rheumatologist about triggers and autoimmune disease and the correlation between the two. As I started to think about distinctive stressors and the many traumatic medical emergencies that had happened to me since I was a child, I started to see some patterns emerge. In my research, I saw some of those patterns confirmed.

Many in medical research believe there are a few elements that need to be present for a person's immune system to potentially turn against itself—which is, in essence, what autoimmune disease does. Among these necessary elements are

- a person's genetic makeup and predispositions,[3]
- the ways in which hormones affect the body[4] (particularly estrogen), and
- environmental factors . . . or triggers.

Medical research has identified numerous triggers linked to a wide variety of autoimmune diseases, thanks to ongoing research. For example, systemic sclerosis has been linked to exposure to silica dust (often seen in people who work in mining, construction, or farming);[5] exposure to sunlight and other ultraviolet radiation has been associated with juvenile dermatomyositis;[6] and certain pesticides have been connected to rheumatoid arthritis in farmworkers, particularly men.[7] Additional autoimmune disease triggers that are the subject of research include infections, exhaustion, pregnancy, surgery, injury, physical harm, trauma, and high levels of stress, just to name a few.[8]

A medical student at heart, I began to wade through the research. Eventually, I came to define a trigger as anything that influences the immune system, causing it to not work at an optimal level and therefore potentially leaving it susceptible for something in the body to go haywire.

The theory is, introduce a trigger to someone with specific genetic predispositions and certain hormone levels (depending on the disease) or environmental factors, and the result may be a faulty rewiring of cells that were once designed to protect the body *into* cells that instead wage an attack on the body's own tissues and organs.

With nothing but time on my hands, I mentally reviewed the symptoms exhibited in my body following the vehicular event: fever, pain, fatigue, rash, and mouth sores, just to name a few. In the conversation with the rheumatologist, those symptoms were neatly boxed up as the aftermath of my physical injury and trauma triggers. And while being hit by the truck was the trigger that opened the autoimmunity floodgates, in that very moment I gained clarity on the fact that these symptoms *didn't* just show themselves for the first time in my life, but rather they showed themselves for the first time in my life *all at once.*

My mind reeling with different memories, I scooted my body toward the head of my bed and adjusted the pillows behind me so my back had more support. While gingerly trying to reach for a pen and legal pad off of my nightstand, I shouted, "Mom! I need to speak to you! Mom? Ma!" (yes, what others would perceive as shouting, because "shouting" is the baseline level conversational sound in our Italian home).

She ran in with a worried look, as though she expected I'd hurt myself. "Sorry, Mom. I just thought of something, and I had to talk to you, like right now!" As I started writing notes on yellow legal paper, I continued. "So we both know I haven't been healthy since I was young. There was always something happening, right? My health has always been an issue, basically since I was a baby, yet no one could put their finger on it. It was always just, I was 'delicate' or a 'sickly child.' . . . But these symptoms I had in the hospital, I've had them before . . ."

Mom gently pushed against the soles of my feet, signaling for me to move them over and make space for her on the bed. We stared at one another, quietly recounting past health events. "You were always in so much pain growing up," she recalled. "What if it was lupus pain that entire time, and here I was telling you it was growing pains?"

"Mom, there was no way for you to know I had lupus! Even the doctors were clueless. But you are right, I remember the pain in my arms and hands. And rashes after being in the sun, or how tired I was as a child while all of my friends were outside playing. I was the only one in my group of friends who needed naps every single day!"

We created a timeline using the legal pad and made a list of major health symptoms or seasons that stuck out in our minds. While I struggled with allergies and asthma since birth (both intimately tied to the immune system), one particular event on the timeline stood out as a noticeable downturn in my already rocky health. When I was eight, I came down with a severe case of Coxsackie virus during summer camp. I had an extremely high fever for weeks, broke out in dozens of sores in my mouth and nose, experienced extreme weakness to the point where I couldn't walk, and was hospitalized for dehydration. My body was never the same afterward.

From this (perhaps) minitrigger, I struggled with sporadic mouth and nose sores and random fevers. It was also during my teen and young adult years that strange rashes, fatigue, and excruciating body pain showed up, but I never connected any of the dots until now.

Add all of this to recurrent bronchitis and pneumonia infections from asthma and allergies, and I was literally in the doctor's office almost monthly throughout my childhood. "Mom, with all the doctors I saw, how did no doctor see these symptoms as a part of something bigger?"

The story of living years with undiagnosed symptoms of autoimmune disease and not understanding the underlying cause isn't unique. And many parents, children, victims of trauma, and health-challenged individuals struggle for years to put the pieces of a puzzle together that never quite seem to fit.

Autoimmune diseases are tricky and difficult to diagnose. It also doesn't help the "trying to determine a diagnosis" situation when there are over one hundred types of autoimmune diseases, according to the American Autoimmune Related Diseases Association (AARDA).[9] In addition, many symptoms from one autoimmune disease can overlap with another, building more layers of difficulty when it comes to receiving a clear and accurate diagnosis. Currently, AARDA states that the average amount of time it takes a patient to receive a correct autoimmune diagnosis is three or more years—with the individual seeing an average of four or more physicians during that period.[10] With lupus, organizations like the Lupus Foundation of America estimate it takes an average of *six* years and at least four physicians to get an accurate lupus diagnosis, with—sit down for this one—some surveys reflecting that over 60 percent of people living with lupus stating they received at least one incorrect diagnosis before being accurately diagnosed.[11]

Lupus is often called the "great mimicker." Lupus symptoms imitate those seen in many other diseases, and these symptoms typically come and go, so they aren't always seen by physicians on the day of your visit—as was the case with my own story. For most of us, it can be a challenging road to a firm diagnosis. And what many people diagnosed with chronic illness share, myself included, is there is also often a long period of emotional suffering alongside the physical issues as individuals search for a correct diagnosis.

By my early teens, I accepted that I was different from my friends when it came to my health. My health issues caused me to miss school often, to spend time in doctors' offices, and I was among the few kids I knew at my school who carried around all of their medications in their backpack every single day. A lot of the time, I also looked gaunt and pale, with dark black circles under my eyes and bones protruding from my skinny frame—let's just say this didn't do much for my social life or my romantic life as I matured.

Creating the timeline with my mother caused different levels of distress for both of us. Why was I never tested for lupus . . . or any other autoimmune disease, for that matter? For those who have suffered for years with strange symptoms, finally getting a concrete diagnosis also brings with it a flood of emotions. There is relief in finally having an answer to the bizarre symptoms that have plagued us, but along with the relief can come feelings of resentment—as the suffering has gone on for far too many years and negatively impacted crucial years of socialization, education, employment, and relationships.

Many of us living in the prediagnosis state of sporadic symptoms—which often do not present at the same time—also live with the common reality of not being taken seriously. This is especially true if you are a woman. For years, my and my mom's concerns about my body never fully stabilizing after the Coxsackie incident were met with symptoms being downplayed and fevers, rashes, and fatigue being brushed off as me just having a fragile immune system since early childhood. Doctors would respond that I "seemed" to be adapting to my limitations (because children are "stronger than we think they are"—don't even get me started on that comment from one of my former doctors). While I do agree that children are resilient in their own right, I also think medical experts who don't dig deeper when young patients are continually suffering and who offer no support and no answers—except for pat comments on resiliency—need to be called out and challenged.

When it comes to health concerns, research highlights the heartbreaking reality that women are not as likely as men to have their health concerns addressed appropriately and taken as seriously by doctors. Studies show that women are half as likely as men to receive pain medication during the first three days after surgery and are forced to wait longer periods of time for medication as compared to men; plus, when being treated for similar issues in an emergency room, women are seven times more likely than men to be misdiagnosed in the midst of a heart attack.[12]

The inherent sexism and medical-related gender biases have gone on far too long and have yet to be addressed in a significant way by the medical community.

Partially, this is the result of long-standing medical and disease concepts originally formulated based on the physiology of men (women were not legally allowed to participate in medical/clinical research studies until the passing of the NIH Revitalization Act of 1993, which established the inclusion of women and minorities in clinical research after a 1977 FDA guideline banning most women of childbearing age from medical research)[13] combined with an irrational, long-held stereotype in the medical community that women are melodramatic when it comes to voicing their health concerns and symptoms (hence the catchall term *female hysteria*, which basically mislabeled women's physical health concerns as purely psychological)[14]. These gender disparities mean that when women raise health issues, the bias against women in the health care system not only harms each individual diagnosis but especially harms the lupus and other immune-compromised communities (in which the majority of patients are female) in which the already-difficult process of correct diagnosis is exponentially devastating.

Many women have a keen intuition when it comes to their body and their baseline. They are able to recognize issues early when something seems awry. So why are our observations regarding unusual symptoms and health patterns being discounted by so many doctors so that we not only *do not get* the dignity of a correct diagnosis, but we are often made to doubt our own intuition and shy away from speaking up for ourselves?[15] The gaslighting that is accepted as part of traditional medical communities is harmful and prevents countless people from receiving the help they desperately need.

Why must we fight so hard just for someone in the medical community—whose commitment is to help people with health challenges—to listen to us?

The more I ruminated on a lifetime of medical treatment that not only didn't seriously address my health issues but also caused added loss, worry, pain, social stigma, and shame, the angrier I became.

"Come on, your wheels are spinning. You need to get away from the four walls of this room and sit with us while Grandma makes dinner." I didn't reject the invitation, as the smell of garlic began to fill the air. While I was too sick to stand near the oven and countertop to help my grandmother prepare her stuffed artichokes, being in the kitchen had always been my comfort. As I sat at the table, I knew immediately that returning to the kitchen and moving forward with my life in general was something I needed to force myself to do, regardless of my feelings of despair for systems that failed me or the impatience I had around my slow progress. As my grandmother meticulously filled each artichoke leaf with her homemade stuffing, she glanced in my direction, smiling, and gave me a wink. "I miss my helper," she whispered.

"I've missed you too, Grandma."

I doodled on the side edge of the legal pad that came along for the trip into the kitchen and looked at my mother for some time before questioning, "So how am I supposed to reconcile feeling angry that my health problems were discounted for so long while also resting in this feeling of gratitude to God that I finally have a diagnosis and survived a potentially deadly experience?" My grandmother and mother had different responses to the question, and the more deeply we engaged in conversation, the more of a revelation I had.

Part of this revelation involved the dangers of the mind jumping back and forth between two conflicting emotions and thoughts. These two things couldn't coexist in my mind or my heart in an eternal game of Ping-Pong. That would only lead me to a kind of restless double mind. I could focus on my anger and anxiety about what happened to me in the past. I could acknowledge and feel the true anger that was there but refuse to "live there." And I could trust in what I'd known to this point: the love and wisdom of God and my current situation. My mom, of course, dug out her ever-present Bible and talked about the letter from James.

The letter is about difficulties and challenges in life. Depending on how we respond, these challenges can produce endurance and shape our character. She explained that a good barometer of our character is how we react and express ourselves when under pressure or when we feel anger. Most of us can use some work in this area. But I *really needed* some work here. As she explained it, God wants our character to be formed and resilience to grow, and it's through challenges we face that our character develops more and more into wholeness. We aren't made whole when we blame. We aren't experiencing joy in its fullness when we refuse to believe God can still do amazing things no matter our suffering and no matter our difficult circumstances.

At the end of the day, she said, we need to decide which "mind" we will choose to spend time with, which one will win out. I could work to right the wrongs that occurred in the world, but to live in anger and resentment was no way to right those wrongs.

To truly love myself and put my physical and mental health first, to truly right those wrongs, I would need to acknowledge that, yes, while I was ignored and discounted for years by the medical community, to continue to hold on to the harm done to me, to sit in anger, would destroy me. That was giving others and their actions power over my life. And I didn't want to allow anyone else destructive power. In fact, didn't it make sense to take that harm and anger and mistreatment and use it to ensure no other woman would have to experience the heartbreak of not knowing what was going wrong inside her body?

There was a hope and peace I could choose, the way that Job kept choosing to look toward an honest relationship with God no matter how unsure he was about the losses or how difficult the path forward looked—or even whether he saw a way forward. Job prayed for wisdom. He talked to God and believed that God would give it generously.

That night as I headed back to bed, after the wisdom of the kitchen and the gift of the shared meal, I cried again, asking the Creator to help me let go of the anger I was holding on to due to the mistakes the medical community had made. To let go of the physical and emotional pain it caused me. This was a tough one for me. The medical personnel who didn't recognize that something was wrong, who refused to listen to my concerns and my mother's concerns all those years—could I forgive them? Could I forgive the person who hit me with their truck? As I asked myself these questions, I also understood that each time I thought about them as people to blame, I felt like I was being poisoned. The harm and poison were there. But I didn't want to keep drinking the poison. Those injustices could only bring more harm if I focused on them. I envisioned a cloud of blackness being wiped away into a clean, vibrant slate full of bright light while I prayed, asking God to purify my heart and mind.

Rather than being distracted constantly by something from the past, shifting between an anger that was harming me and being of a double mind, I wanted to have feet firmly on the ground.

I also asked for wisdom about the new realities of my current situation. I understood my entire life had changed, and I needed guidance to discover this "new" me whose character was being shaped through each new challenge.

As I wiped my wet cheeks with my pajama sleeves, I said, "God, anything else in me that needs to go, that's preventing me from growing my faith and my character, I'm handing it over—I don't want to carry this pain and anger and hurt anymore. My mom tells me you are in the business of restoring fractured people and making them whole. I just want you to know I'm ready to see us create something beautiful out of all of these broken pieces."

RECIPE

Strawberry Cacao Oat Smoothie

Prep/Blend Time: 5 minutes
Method: Blender
Yield: 1 serving

Sometimes, when we feel exhausted, fractured, in the hard work of seeking wholeness, a simple smoothie like this—delicious and quick and easy to prepare—can offer just the right break, give just the right boost. This is one of my favorite recipes, and depending on what type of milk and yogurt alternative you use, you can pack plenty of protein into this drink. I also add

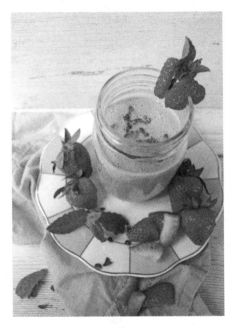

unflavored collagen powder to increase the protein content, plus collagen powder is great for your skin, hair, and even gut health. Last, the alkalinity and bitterness of the cacao nibs really even out the sweetness of the strawberries to make the perfect combination. If you *really* like your smoothies extra sweet, you can also add a teaspoon of honey or maple syrup to this recipe.

INGREDIENTS

½ cup rolled oats
½ cup milk or milk alternative
One 5.3-ounce container of strawberry yogurt (or yogurt
    alternative)
1 cup fresh strawberries, stems removed
½ teaspoon vanilla extract
1 tablespoon of your favorite collagen powder (I use Further Food),
    optional
1 teaspoon cacao nibs

Optional
Honey or maple syrup, if you prefer really sweet smoothies

Add your oats to the blender, cover, and use the "grind" button for 10–15 seconds until the oats are ground into more of a flour texture. Next, add milk, yogurt, strawberries, vanilla extract, and collagen powder. Switch back to blend and blend ingredients well. Last, add cacao nibs and blend for another 10 seconds. If you prefer a thinner smoothie, you can add another ¼ cup milk. If you prefer a thicker smoothie, add more fruit. Drink immediately, and if you prefer, serve over ice. Enjoy!

SIX

Seasons of Recalibration

Faith doesn't always mean that God changes your situation. Sometimes it means God changes you.
—Pastor Steven Furtick (adapted)

Back in 1967, two psychiatrists, Thomas Holmes and Richard Rahe, examined how life stressors could contribute to changes in a person's physical health. To support the study, they created the now-renowned Holmes and Rahe Stress Scale. The scale lists forty-three life events known to cause some level of stress to the human body. These life events range from those creating major stress on the body (the death of a spouse, listed as number one) to those creating minor stress on the body (like getting a ticket for a minor traffic violation, such as jaywalking, listed as number forty-three on the scale). At number six on the scale is experiencing personal illness or injury, just behind death of a spouse / death of a family member, divorce, separation from a partner, or imprisonment.

It's no secret that illness can turn our world upside down. If we are diagnosed with a chronic and incurable illness, it isn't uncommon to meet the diagnosis with shock or denial or disconnection from reality for a period of time. This is something our bodies and minds do and may serve as a protective mechanism helping us to continue functioning without a complete meltdown. In time, as we slowly move away from the shock and begin wading through the stages of grief—from denial and anger to bargaining and then depression—we eventually get to a place where we begin to process the situation and absorb the related information. Once we are able to start processing information, we can work toward building something that will affect every aspect of our life moving forward, and that stage is *acceptance*, as we face what has now become a part of our life.

Now, I'm not saying we have to run with wide open arms to acceptance of an illness shortly after being diagnosed. But ignoring it or fighting it with every fiber of our being won't help us bring *any* level of healing to our heart, body, or soul in the long term. It's important to remember that when we are handed a diagnosis, this is a time we *need* healing in these areas. To delay the healing is to further harm ourselves. Eventually, we have to make a decision. You may choose to live in denial of the diagnosis and denial that anything in your life has changed, which will lead to continual turmoil in your heart and mind. Or you can recognize that *elements* of your life have changed.

The challenging part here is separating those elements of our identity that have changed from those that are constants, keeping our overall identity intact. While we recognize that an illness may limit things like mobility, stamina, different activities, or our social lives, it *never* gets to take away the person God created us to be, with our dreams, our hopes, our life story, our unique personality, our sense of humor, our warm heart, our kindness, and our purpose. We have the opportunity to actively make the decision to firmly hold on to these things—and even allow them to flourish—with God's help, despite what any illness can throw at us.

After a rocky and anger-filled early response to my lupus diagnosis, I began to slowly come to terms with it. I came to the realization that I could *discover* who I was becoming in this new chapter of my life, or I could deny who I was becoming—but I wouldn't have the energy or mental capacity to do both.

One choice meant that a new path would open up for me, providing a breakthrough where I was given the opportunity and the freedom to learn where God was leading me in each new day—and how God was going to work in my heart and refine me through this discovery process.

The other path of resistance and denial meant being rigid and difficult. Rejecting this new life meant there would be constant turmoil, because that meant rejecting new life experiences that came through this new situation while I was focused on only comparing myself to what used to be. Later, my husband and I would call the latter path "The Town of Used To"—the place those with chronic illness travel to at times when comparing their new life to their old, illness-free life. This choice, this trip, is no holiday. In fact, this type of travel never feels like a peaceful, relaxing vacation. Instead, "The Town of Used To" leaves you defeated, unrested, and exhausted in the constant fight *against* something rather than *for* something.

After a few short visits to "Used To," I decided to refuse to travel back to this town. Discovery and new life seemed so much more appealing to my soul than the life-draining "what was" and "what should be."

As I prayed, listened, and leaned into the questions of my new life and the struggles of my heart, God placed in me a deep desire to discover this "new" me. As I began to understand more about God in prayer and the silence of listening, I also began to learn more about myself. And part of this discovery for me was leaning into my joy of reading and learning. While I was no longer studying for nursing, I began to study and research lupus and chronic illness more generally, understanding more about these new elements in my life. I'm an information junkie, and at the time, the internet was in its early days, so I returned to one of my favorite places—the library. Growing up, Grandma, Bogey (Grandpa), and I would go to the library every Saturday at 9 a.m. Bogey would lose himself in the row of books that held carpentry and woodworking titles, while Grandma veered toward romance, history, and biographies. She would check out six to seven books each week and finish them by the following Saturday. And I would be free to roam and choose my set of books for the week.

With my new physical limitations, Mom drove Grandma and me to the library each week. She'd push me up and down aisle after aisle in my wheelchair as I grabbed hold of any book I could find on lupus, autoimmune disease, food, and diet. The pickings were slim. But I began to build a foundation of knowledge.

Ever since I was a child, I've had a fascination with the human body, hence my desire to become a nurse. After the return from the hospital, I would spend hours reading and lying in bed, considering how food and herbs play a role in the healing or rebuilding process.

As I considered all the ways God had become my soul nourishment in the spiritual sense, I wondered what kind of nourishment my body needed: how rehab, exercise, rest, and the foods I consumed were all elements of the physical nourishment my body longed for. Looking at the foods I was eating, I began to ask questions. Was I choosing the right foods—ingredients that best suited my body's needs in this moment? How best could my body create the energy it needed to repair itself—to absorb the many required nutrients for the billions of biological processes that happen in my body daily? What was it that my body desperately needed?

Unfortunately, back then, there was a dearth of information, research, and personal testimonies on how certain foods and diet types influenced autoimmune symptoms. And don't get me started on gut health and how that played into immunity—when I'd mention it at that time, I was often met with blank stares. And while some in the medical field took gut health seriously, most doctors looked at me like I was loony tunes. It was 2001 and the internet suffered from limited information, the majority of which was from the Western medicine community that suffered from antiquated thinking when it came to the role of diet in our physical health. (Thank God, times have changed!) So knowing there was something more to learn and having understood I had met with healing elements in my grandmother's kitchen, I turned to books, research, and appointments with a nutritionist, all the while experimenting with foods and nutritional concepts to find some answers.

As I continued to read, experiment, and ask questions, I found a community of thinkers and nontraditional practitioners who introduced me to the role of food and herbs and how they can impact inflammation within the body of someone with an inflammatory disease like lupus. I began learning about the gut, how intimately it is tied to the immune system, and how an unbalanced biome or leaky gut can cause a chain reaction of issues within the body as it reacts to ingested food. I was introduced to fasting, allergy and sensitivity testing, juicing, and the role of herbs and functional medicine and how along with Western medicine, I could create an all-encompassing protocol for my body. And part of this protocol was finding my new food "normal" as I learned which foods caused allergic reactions and which foods I was sensitive to or in fact aggravated lupus symptoms.

The more I read, the more I learned, and the more I learned, the more my mind was fed and both my physical and spiritual appetites grew. For the first time in so many months, I noticed a feeling that had been so distant, a feeling I believed would never come again—excitement. Along with the excitement came an overwhelming desire to get back into the kitchen, to wash fresh vegetables and fruits and herbs and create something life giving with them for my body. I wanted to spread open a ripe pomegranate, to see its bright-red juice running over my hands and wrists as I felt its crisp arils between my fingers. I needed to hear the sound of fresh garlic and diced onions sizzling as they are sautéed in olive oil, their aroma filling the home. I wanted to experiment with different grains and flours and breads—those full of nutrients, like millet, buckwheat, oat, and amaranth—and feel the dough spread between my fingers as I kneaded it and watched it come to life. I wanted to find the most nutritious foods possible and introduce them all into my broken body. I wanted my body to soak up every droplet of nutrition from only the best foods so it could have the greatest chance of making it through this battle.

And so my return to the kitchen took flight.

The first few weeks I was officially back in the kitchen were both exhilarating and draining. As if we never missed a beat, we jumped right back into stuffing artichokes, boiling down escarole, peeling potatoes, and baking fresh apples. All of my senses were once again engaged, a flood of emotions mixed with the contentedness of being back with my grandmother, and it felt life-giving and almost intoxicating.

I didn't think it was possible, but Grandma may have been even more excited than I was. We fell back into our rhythm so quickly, there were moments when it seemed like I never left. Like the old Marisa still existed. Sometimes the only thing that brought me back to reality in those moments of joy was the sudden hit of exhaustion. Just fifteen to twenty minutes on my feet—even with my walker—brought shattering fatigue that sent me straight to my room. At first the fatigue sort of felt like a punishment. I wrestled with the fact that my mind was spinning and wanted to do a million things, but my body was apparently still on strike. In those moments I took advantage of the mental energy I experienced and returned to one of my very first loves—writing. I've filled notebooks and journals with notes, stats, and diagrams on everything from the pathophysiology of the inflammatory cascade in the body and how people with autoimmune disease need to recognize flare triggers to how herbs like ginger, holy basil, rosemary, and turmeric can reduce pain and inflammation in the body.

I also started writing down food experiments and differences in body energy in my daily calendar planner. Journaling eventually offered a storehouse of invaluable data that I'd return to over the next two decades. Each day I kept notes on how much I slept and napped, my pain levels, every item of food ingested, medications and supplements taken, any stressors (good and bad) experienced, my menstrual cycle, and reactions to being in the sun. These life event notes also included specific details of how my body was affected by different foods, herbs, medicines, or supplements. While other people I knew were filling their calendar planners with school and work schedules, social and evening events, and travel plans, I filled mine with little nuggets of gold that—while I didn't know it at the time—would later help me build a treasure trove of wisdom for how to live my best life for my body's needs.

As I journaled the details, I also continued to pray, asking God to help me see the good in this situation, to see what God was doing. For many of us who deal with immune issues or trauma to the body, one ongoing challenge we meet is that the mind can release thoughts that quickly go in unhealthy directions when we are stationary for a long period of time due to illness or injury. When I was able to stay focused on the good, I was less overwhelmed by the physical pain or the physical limitations I was dealing with.

You may know personally how hard it is to see the good in anything when you are in excruciating pain; sometimes the mental struggle of it all seems more challenging than the actual physical pain itself. Slowly, I started to see this time of recovery as a quiet season of discovery, where I was stripped from all of the distractions once filling my life. And in this quiet space, not only did my love for food return, but so did my love for writing. In the chaos that was my life before being hit—college, working full time, helping care for my grandmother, dating, studying, and having a social life—I never made time for writing, even though I always "wanted" to. I got wrapped up in the excuses and busy-ness of life and lost that part of myself. This new season now brought the opportunity. Not only did I begin journaling and writing about the research, but I began to write poems, prayers, and love notes to God; letters in response to newspaper op-eds; wish lists for the future. My heart poured out on paper. Soon, I was thanking God for this opportunity—even though I wasn't thrilled about the trauma to my body. I was beginning to glimpse how a loving God was using the situation to help me rediscover myself. And in that, my level of joy continued to increase. And while my initial reaction to everything that happened to me was to fight it tooth and nail, I began to recognize that through a budding faith, I was learning to acclimate and discover new joys.

Author Sherri Mandell shares that "in every trauma, there is a shattering and an opportunity for rebirth." I couldn't agree more, and with that rebirth, I feel there is freedom. Everyone living with chronic illness will—at some point—come to the realization that the higher your ability to adapt to the changes happening in your body and to changes in your overall life, the more peace and overall freedom you will have. It may sound strange to list *freedom* as a possible aftereffect of chronic illness, but think of it this way: Chronic illness is basically waging a war on our physical body, which often means there's a war raging within, mentally. If we focus solely on the illness and what it is taking away from us, we are losing the war and ourselves in the midst of it. But when we spiritually grow, when we learn to adapt, something shifts.

Adapting for us means changing in a variety of ways that allow us to deal with our new circumstances—and illness sure does bring about a wild set of new circumstances. Adapting offers us freedom. Rather than giving all of our power over to the illness, illness instead follows *our* lead.

In the very origin of the word *adapt*, the Proto-Indo-European *ap* means to "take" or "grasp." When I first learned about this word's roots, I had an incredibly vivid vision of grabbing this destructive entity that was lupus, my hand acting as a bridle. Without me taking hold of it, this entity was like a whirlwind completely whipping up noise around me. But instead of letting it swirl around me, clouding my ability to see what was in front of me—what was my future—I needed to let go of my fear of the whirlwind, constrain it, and take control. I needed to adapt.

Chronic illness asks all of us to adapt.

Yes, lupus literally cost me not only a nursing career but the loss of what I felt I was put on the earth to do. After spending years as a chemistry major and busting my tail to keep a 4.0 while working full time so I could receive scholarships, it ended. I had my pity party—my party of one. And I fully allowed myself to feel the hurt and pain in watching a career slip through my fingers so quickly, something I worked so incredibly hard for. What were my choices moving forward? I could play the same tape over and over for the rest of my life: "I was supposed to be a nurse, but since that was taken away, I'm not going to be able to fulfill my dreams." Or I could pull on my big-girl panties and say, "Okay, God, what is next? A hundred nails were put into that door that shut with a bang, but I know you gave me other gifts and talents. So what now? That longing in me to be of service, to help others heal is still strong. What can that look like now?"

When I think of people who have been models for me of living and thriving despite devastating trauma and illness, two incredible human beings come to mind. One woman I utterly adore and look up to in so many ways—as our life situations have so many similarities—is Frida Kahlo. When she was eighteen, she was in a vehicular accident that literally sent a handrail piercing through her back and out through her pelvis. As if her spinal and pelvic fractures weren't enough, her foot was crushed, her ribs were broken, and she had numerous breaks in her leg and collarbone. And this is after surviving polio! Even with the pain I endured, I couldn't imagine her pain—plus, she survived the life-altering event in 1925, during a time the medical field still had few surgical resources, therapies, or medications. Could Frida have lain in bed for the rest of her life, hindered by her suffering, and foregoing the dreams she held? She sure could. With injuries so severe, anyone would have been hard pressed to argue that she needed to "get up and get moving and get on" with her life. But even with all of her physical challenges, Frida had the wisdom at her young age to let the experience become the inspiration that would propel her to be one of history's most famous female artists. And where did she create the majority of her paintings? From her bed! Incorporating her own experiences with mental anguish and the brokenness of her physical body, she began to pour out her talents onto a canvas rigged to fit over her in bed. She refused to let what would be a lifetime of limitations keep her from fulfilling her purpose.

Another inspiration for me is the transformation that happened in the life of Joni Erickson Tada. When she was just seventeen, she became a quadriplegic after a diving accident in the Chesapeake Bay. Paralyzed from the shoulders down, she struggled with rage, suicidal thoughts, depression, and questioning her faith in God. As she sought to reconcile those things, she began to paint, using a paintbrush placed in between her teeth. She began a transformational journey that led her to create and sell her paintings, as well as write over forty-five books. Here's a woman with technically no use of her arms writing books, creating artwork, becoming a recording artist, and founding one of the largest Christian ministries that helps others deal with disability—Joni and Friends. When she was once asked what her suffering has taught her, she said, "I'd say it's the textbook that teaches me who I really am. Suffering keeps knocking me off my pedestal of pride."[1]

Fabulous Finds

Make a Commitment

Make a commitment. #SpeakLife over yourself each day, even if it is only for a minute or two. And even if it feels awkward or uncomfortable. Generously pour love onto yourself, reminding yourself that you are loved, beautiful, unique, valuable, talented, and a warrior.

It's that same passion and refusal to let their talents be wasted by tragedy in people like Joni and Frida that runs through the veins of countless men and women today who have adapted due to their chronic illness journey. Over the years I've met some amazing men and women who have lost everything—finances, relationships, independence, mobility, their careers, and so on— only to rebuild a foundation and flourish. They've gone on to become inspirational health advocates and public speakers, prolific authors, artists making the world a more adapted place for people with disabilities or illness, nonprofit founders, YouTube educators, and more—the opportunities are endless!

Wherever you are on this journey, you'll come to the realization that this life-changing event or diagnosis you went through is forever going to be a defining point in your life. And you'll start to remember that you have a range of choices other than letting this trauma or illness or injury or event become your sole definition—your identity—that follows you around like a gray cloud; you can shift focus to recapturing dreams, envisioning new directions, seeing the one who created you, and looking with faith to understand your purpose and definition.

Challenging seasons are ones that call for recalibration. They are opportunities to rediscover ourselves and, with God's help, take inventory of who we truly are, who we want to become, and how we can use the talents and gifts we have been given. Because, trust me—there are many. And when we are reminded of our definition, of who we truly are in God's eyes—not defined by our illness or trauma—we learn a new definition, and we are set free.

All throughout scripture are God's promises of that definition. We are

- loved and chosen by God,
- accepted,
- wonderfully made,
- gifted and talented,
- valuable and valued,
- never alone or forsaken,
- transformed, and
- set free.

It was in learning who God says I am *and* repeating it to myself that I finally started to believe I was valued, gifted, free. And it didn't happen overnight, or even over months. For a long time, I felt less than. But slowly I began to feel a change in me, from the time I was injured and diagnosed to when I began to feel excitement, empowerment, and strength. My career path had changed, but my mission to educate myself and understand how all that I learned might be a vehicle for not only my own change and strength but those of others as well was now at the forefront of my mind.

Healthy Cranberry Orange Breakfast Bread

Prep Time: 15 minutes
Cook Time: 15 minutes
Method: Stovetop, oven, and electric hand mixer
Yield: 8 servings

Breakfast is by far my favorite meal, and I prefer to start my day off with something hearty and filling rather than something too sweet. This cranberry orange bread has healthy ingredients, and the dried cranberries and honey give it just the kick it needs. While I use oat flour in my recipe, you can play around with coconut, almond, or gluten-free varieties depending on your dietary needs. You can also swap out the dried cranberries for another type of dried fruit, but keep the ratio the same. I start many of my days with some version of this bread and a hot cup of cinnamon and clove tea. You can heat up a slice in a toaster oven in the morning and put a little butter or butter

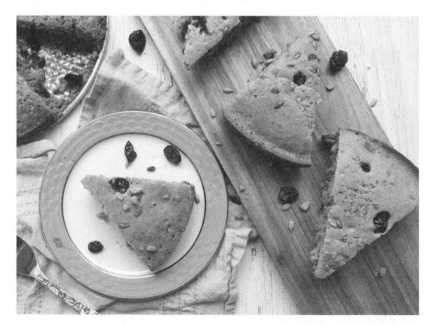

alternative on it, or if you have a sweet tooth, some powdered sugar works well too!

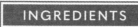

INGREDIENTS

¼ cup melted butter or coconut oil, plus extra to grease the pan
1½ cups oat flour (or try almond, coconut, or gluten-free)
½ teaspoon baking soda
1 teaspoon ground flaxseed
¼ teaspoon salt
4 large eggs
5 tablespoons honey (you could also use maple syrup or agave syrup)
1 large orange, broken down into:
    1–2 teaspoons grated orange zest and ⅓ cup fresh orange juice
1 tablespoon vanilla extract
¾ cup dried cranberries (Craisins), with a little extra for topping
⅓ cup shelled sunflower seeds, with a little extra for topping
One 9-inch springform pan

Optional Toppings
Butter or butter alternative spread on it after lightly toasting it
Powdered sugar sprinkled over it

Preheat your oven to 350°F. Melt your butter or coconut oil on the stovetop and take off the heat when finished. Grease a 9-inch springform or round cake pan very well. Sift the oat flour and baking soda into a large bowl, then add the ground flaxseed and salt and stir well with a spoon until mixed. In a separate bowl, combine the eggs, honey, melted butter/oil, grated orange zest, fresh orange juice, and vanilla extract using a whisk.

Next, slowly pour the wet ingredient mixture into the dry ingredient bowl and mix thoroughly with an electric hand mixer. Last, sprinkle in your dried cranberries and sunflower seeds slowly, folding in a little at a time. Pour the mixture into your greased pan and spread evenly. At this point, I like to take a few extra dried cranberries and sunflower seeds and sprinkle on the top for aesthetic reasons. Bake for 15 minutes or until the outside is light golden brown and a fork or toothpick in the center comes out clean. Remove from oven and let it cool before removing from the pan. If desired, serve with a smear of butter on top or sprinkled powdered sugar.

SEVEN

Our Uniquely Designed Purpose

*The most dangerous thing in the
world is to have no purpose.*
—Bishop T. D. Jakes

I f you've ever had everything seemingly crumbling around you, placing you in the center of fiery ruins, so to speak, eventually it's likely that you will ask, Can I—and how do I—rebuild from here? And what will my newly rebuilt life look like moving forward? When we meet a season of radical change due to illness or injury or one of the million other life-altering events that can occur, we contemplate how our new circumstances will intersect with every area of our lives. We might question if we will have to change careers, alter a current college path, or completely forego working for a season. We'll consider the effects the illness or injury will have on our relationships—from our romantic relationships to our platonic friendships. Our thoughts will likely swing wildly in a variety of directions: *Will my partner and spouse stay with me if my level of independence* (read: dependence) *changes? Will they be able to handle the emotional and physical challenges this disease could bring into our life together* (because it will in fact bring challenges)*?*

For those who are single, wondering how illness or trauma or injury will affect new dating experiences is also common. Some may wonder about disclosing a diagnosis in a new relationship. And if not immediately, *when* should they know? And how do you tell them? And for those who have children, how does that trauma or illness affect their lives? Or what might it mean about potentially having children in the future, if that's even a possibility? All of these things are a lot to reconcile on top of physically and emotionally coming to terms with a new illness, loss, or trauma in your life. Is it any wonder we can sometimes feel so completely overwhelmed?

The truth of the matter is, literally every single aspect of our life—including those in closest relationship to us—will change when something like illness is thrown into the mix.

Upon my arrival home from the hospital, there was no aspect of my life that was unchanged. And while there was no doubt in my mind that God had seen me through getting hit by the truck and the diagnosis, as I looked toward the future, I wanted to know the reason *why* I survived a trauma that even the trauma surgeon working on me didn't expect me to survive when I first arrived at the hospital. I also desperately wanted to know, *God, what is the purpose in all that's taking place?*

As I moved through stages of grief, as I turned a corner on the anger and resentment at losing my career and independence as a result of an event that was just a few seconds in the making and a lifetime requiring my response, I started to consider that maybe my purpose for being alive *wasn't* in being a nurse after all—and trust me, this wasn't easy to come to terms with. In fact, there was a lot of anger I needed to work through when it came to saying goodbye to this dream. Ever since I was young, I thought that nursing would be the best, most direct, and fitting path for helping and serving people. *How could I have gotten my life's path so wrong?* I wondered.

As I began to question why God gave me an innate desire for a career that I couldn't fulfill, I wondered if there was something in that career path, that hope, that I was still meant for. What if there was a way I could still use my desire to help people, but in a different way? What would that look like in my current state? And what could that look like moving forward?

Even with all the changes, I realized that I was the one who was surprised, confused, angry, detoured. But I also had the sense that everything that transpired wasn't a surprise for God. I thought back to what I'd learned about the story of Job—where none of the events, none of the questions, came as a surprise to God. Despite unexpected detours and our worst losses, God has a design. God isn't surprised when we become sick or experience something life shattering. God doesn't shape us in our mother's bellies and then get stymied by the curveball of a chronic illness or a trauma with long-lasting repercussions.

To keep the baseball metaphor, when there's a curveball, the God at bat swings and meets the ball. And doesn't miss.

I realized that while I was the one freaking out and with questions about my carrying out a purpose and plan, I was met time and time again by a God who knocked it out of the park. I was suddenly handed a variety of limitations, but God responded with an infinite variety of options.

Before, I never stood still or quiet long enough to think about anything but the daily rituals in my life and one single goal. Now I was in this slow season of radical change, and that mission kept expanding. My mother would continually speak life and encouragement over me, talking to me about our being beautifully and wonderfully made, formed in personhood and mission, with talents and gifts from the time of the womb. As I listened to her read a psalm about purpose one night, I wondered, *Is there really more for me than being sick? Is there life and purpose for me outside of these four walls of my bedroom?*

I learned that even before that sense of career purpose, there was another purpose. On this life journey, we are created to know God, to be in ongoing communication and relationship, sharing our daily lives with God, and learning to trust the Creator's lead. It was in this ever-blossoming relationship with the Creator that I learned to discover more about my life's purpose. And I learned to trust that God takes my physical and mental abilities, my personality, life experiences, and gifts, and builds something extraordinary—something fabulous—to fulfill the unique purpose given to each one of us.

"We are God's masterpiece," one Bible passage says, and "we can do the good things [God] planned for us long ago" (Ephesians 2:10 NLT).

No accidents, no random ideas, you and I were created to be masterpieces! Long before we ever walked the earth. Before we were born, a plan was forming.

One of the Hebrew prophets, Jeremiah, wrote these words: "For surely I know the plans I have for you, says the Lord, plans for your welfare and not for harm, to give you a future with hope" (Jeremiah 29:11).

There are no Bible verses or promises stating that we won't be met with difficulties and challenges. But there are a variety of statements promising us a hope and future even when the challenges arise. And perhaps the challenge to us when we are met with those statements is, Do you truly believe them? In those awful moments, where we're in a bad headspace and with all the negative things we're telling ourselves, do we cling to the belief that our life is over because X, Y, and Z happened, or can we hold tight, white knuckled, to the hope that we can still live out our purpose despite difficult circumstances?

When we initially meet our limitations, one of the first things we might do is downplay our value to ourselves, to God, to others. We might think, *Well, I can barely function and/or take care of myself, so how can I be of any use to anyone else? I'm just no good.* This thought process can be our first step onto a very slippery slope. And sometimes, as if our own negative self-talk isn't bad enough for us, we get that same harmful message from others too—if we aren't like them or don't meet their expectations. That kind of "less than" judgment from healthy-bodied friends, family, or even strangers can pierce our hearts. If we constantly focus on a medical definition of ourselves, though, we are walking a continuously dangerous line that will never lead to peace. If we continue down this path, we may soon only define ourselves by what happened to us and our medical condition, taking on an illness identity.[1]

We may render ourselves unworthy or inferior—a very dangerous lie to believe.

Reduced to a diagnosis, we downplay our value and gifts. "Marisa," my mom told me one day, "you are not just 'the sick girl with lupus.'" Looking me in the eye, she said, "You are *so* much more than this. And don't diminish yourself—or what God can do—by comparing yourself to others who aren't experiencing exactly what you are going through."

Comparing ourselves to people who have a life journey completely different from ours is a pattern of thinking that quickly takes us away from our own unique destiny. We get so wrapped up in the lives and talents and happenings of someone else that we rob ourselves of recognizing the incredible things that are true about our own lives.

Another way we devalue ourselves while reconciling our future with an illness is by minimizing our role. We believe that our purpose is diminished and that what we have to offer is less than.

My mom, of course, had another set of verses on this: "A body is made up of many parts, and each of them has its own use. That's how it is with us. . . . God has also given each of us different gifts to use. . . . If we can serve others, we should serve. If we can teach, we should teach. If we can encourage others, we should encourage them. If we can give, we should be generous. If we are leaders, we should do our best. If we are good to others, we should do it cheerfully" (Romans 12:4–8 CEV).

Not only was I at a place where I was trying to imagine my life path and what it now looked like, but I was also aware that there were so many ways I might be tempted to diminish my value, my role, my future. I wanted to be intentional in moving forward, in seeing a sense of my purpose, and the way I knew best to discover this was silence, reflection, and prayer.

As I listened, I began to acknowledge that, yes, I had limitations, and I had given up schooling and a career due to health issues, but my gifts, my interests, my talents were all still there. Those didn't take a turn even when events took a turn. Those gifts and talents that were at the very core of my being didn't get ripped away when the whirlwind of life sucked me up and spit me out.

In fact, *nothing* and *no one* can destroy or remove those. Not in me and not in you.

If you are wondering how I found my value and direction even when I was struggling so much with illness, here's what I would tell you: If your life has taken an unexpected turn and you've "forgotten" the person behind the illness, reflect on your youth and the hobbies or activities you loved. Maybe you enjoyed painting or building things, or maybe you gravitated toward gathering people together and planning events or leading an activity.

In these moments, what can you rediscover about yourself?

Maybe you've gotten compliments over the years about a way you are in the world, or about how you treat other people, or about something you excel in. What can you learn from those compliments?

Maybe you are known as someone who is patient and an amazing listener. Perhaps you've been told you're a talented speaker or that when it comes to getting people motivated, you have "the gift." Maybe your words get people fired up. Maybe you are a born leader. Or perhaps like me, you have a knack for bringing a variety of people together through the help of a home-cooked meal, where you listen to them as they pour their hearts out.

Maybe you've forgotten what pulls at your heartstrings. Perhaps you feel a surge of powerful emotions when you see a vulnerable person being taken advantage of, or you feel motivated to create change when you come across injustice in society, or you use your voice for the voiceless. When you begin to reflect on the messages your life has been sharing with you, the gifts you have to share, you might see the hints of your purpose.

Fabulous Finds

Time to Reflect

"If you experience a lack of community, it may mean that you are called upon to build one." —Sherri Mandell

What are you feeling nudged or called to build?

Perhaps you used to help coach your daughter's gymnastics or volleyball team and are frustrated that you do not have the same physical energy to do so at the moment. But maybe you are a great photographer, and instead of coaching, you can sit in the bleachers and take photos that create memories those children can hold onto for a lifetime. Or you might have been a teacher before you became ill, and you miss the joy of explaining something to someone and seeing them grasp a difficult concept for the first time. With technology today, you can literally video record a course or tutor from the privacy of your own home—in your own time frame. Maybe you enjoy writing and want to think creatively about posting work online or have a goal to write a book. Our gifts and talents didn't run for the hills when we were diagnosed with an illness or experienced a trauma. We sometimes just forget—in the flurry of uncertainty—that we need to look at them with fresh eyes as we *adapt* to our new situation.

With long silences, lengthy prayers, adaptation, and attention to the circumstances of my life and the gifts and places in me that ran deeper than illness, I began to see how God had something different planned for me. And that this plan was going to be *different* from everyone else's plan on the planet.

The same goes for you.

The gifts you have and how you use and live into them will look *different* from the plans you may have had and the lives other people live. Let's face it, we live in a society that tends to get judgy when things "look different." But getting caught up in the opinions and judgment of others just takes us away from what *our* purpose *looks like*. When we discover that plan, we understand what purpose God has for *us*—and whatever it "looks" like to other people doesn't matter. They don't get a say in our master plan when they weren't involved in creating the blueprints.

Creamy Mint Cucumber, Tomato, and Feta Salad

Prep Time: 10 minutes
Yield: 4 servings

This creamy salad is the perfect stand-alone snack or side dish to your favorite Mediterranean meal. The fresh mint, fennel, and garlic flavors kick this salad up a notch, and it is one of my favorite dishes to eat as a midday snack. If you prefer topping your salad off with cheese, add a little crumbled feta as the final touch.

INGREDIENTS

2 small cucumbers (skin on or off), diced
3 Roma tomatoes, diced
1 small fennel bulb, greens removed, diced
3 teaspoons fresh mint, chopped
1 heaping teaspoon Italian seasoning
¼ teaspoon Himalayan or sea salt
¼ teaspoon black pepper
¼ cup Greek yogurt or plain yogurt alternative
2 tablespoons olive oil
1 tablespoon apple cider vinegar
2–3 cloves garlic, pressed or minced
Small package feta cheese, optional

In a serving bowl, add the cucumbers, tomatoes, fennel, fresh mint, Italian seasoning, and salt and pepper. Stir to combine. In a separate bowl, add yogurt, olive oil, apple cider vinegar, and garlic. Mix well and then pour over the salad in the serving bowl. Stir until everything is coated. Crumble as much feta on the salad as you prefer—this step is optional, and the salad is delicious even without the cheese added. This salad tastes even better when served cold, so consider covering the bowl with plastic wrap and putting in the refrigerator for 30–60 minutes before serving. Enjoy!

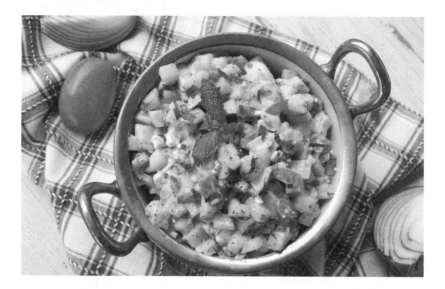

EIGHT

Use Your Voice—
Even If It Shakes

*It only takes one voice, at the right
pitch, to start an avalanche.*

—Dianna Hardy

When we are faced with life-altering events or an unexpected medical diagnosis, not only do our plans for our future change, but so many things also necessarily shift. Our body changes; our immediate goals and needs change. We might meet changes in our work, school, and family life. Our understanding of who we are as a person may also experience a radical shift. But there also may be an incredible evolution that takes place—as I've seen time and time again in the amazing men and women I've come into contact with through the years—when we are suddenly handed the unexpected, even as its specifics and timing are unique to each person.

Some of the people I have encountered, myself included, go through different stages: the pity-party stage, the anger stage, the not-so-smart "I'm going to pretend this isn't happening to me and not take the medicine my doctor gave me" stage (that was me by the way—and an extremely bad idea for your information!), the grief stage, and more. But then, after a variety of stages where you don't even feel like yourself anymore, all of a sudden there is this breakthrough moment. It occurs differently for everyone, but in my experience and from what I've heard most often from others, there seems to be an opening, a juncture, with multiple roads meeting at one center point—like having faith, and experiencing support from family and friends, and coming to terms with what has happened, and innately desiring to hold onto hope, and recognizing there is still this fire inside of you that wants to survive. At one moment they all intersect, and unexpectedly this surge of energy just feels like it is pouring out of you, and if you are like me, you have this sudden urge to shout from the rooftops, "I'm *not* going down! In fact, not only is this disease *not* going to destroy me, but I'm going to show it who's boss . . . all while I somehow make my mark on this world." All of a sudden, you pick up your shield and your sword and you are ready to march onto that battlefield and fight for your life.

And somehow, in that culmination of everything that has been working in your life behind the scenes of the trauma or illness you have been dealing with, your voice finds its way back to you. And you notice it's a little different than it was before. And when you recognize it, it's powerful!

Now, even at this point, you may not know yet how you are going to move forward, but your thinking has made the shift from being the victim of a diagnosis or a traumatic event to being someone who is going to do whatever it takes to not only survive but thrive from here on out.

If you haven't had this breakthrough yet, take courage. Be patient and keep pressing on. No one I've met has had this happen immediately. For me, it literally took years. God had to renew my mind so deeply and so often and help me break unhealthy thinking patterns and anxieties. But I finally reached the point where I wasn't crushed by every little speed bump that lupus brings. For a while there, every little new health surprise brought me a "What now?!" and "Is this going to kill me?" and even a "Why should I even bother doing anything with my life if every week something new is happening with my body?" mentality. These types of thought patterns brought me to some very dark places and threw me off course more times than I want to admit.

Eventually, though, I grew to a place in my life where I could say, "Okay, I've been through worse and survived it, so I am not going to give up just because (insert health disaster here) happened" and "I know God didn't bring me this far to see me fail now. No matter what lupus brings, God's got this."

Somewhere along the way of being hit by the truck and recovering from my injuries only to be hit again with a diagnosis, I lost that spunky, sassy, passionate voice that God gave me. When I finally saw hints of its return, I was elated. In some ways it felt like the "old" me was back—but a stronger, more resilient version.

When I had this breakthrough, I noticed a new, empowered voice began to take root in me. My thinking shifted when it came to addressing all I had to negotiate in life due to lupus. Before, I was completely focused on the new limitations I had from this disease, and these thoughts would get me down, and I would soak my pillow as I sobbed. There were the big limitations, like my inability to physically finish nursing school, and the major change in my energy levels that prevented me from doing simple activities, to smaller limitations like experiencing pain in my hands and arms from chopping vegetables with my grandmother—something I used to be able to do for hours—or missing yet another night out with my friends because, well . . . lupus.

Tired of being constantly frustrated, I slowly began to think of work-arounds I could create that would allow me to still accomplish and enjoy the things I loved most. Rather than giving up on those things I love and narrow-mindedly seeing them as a forever limitation, I began to use my newly found voice within myself. It was sort of a mix between army drill sergeant and loving mother: I'd give myself the gentle reminders I needed that I didn't have to miss out on life altogether because I got handed a big bag of bruised lemons. There were still usable pieces here, but I was going to have to get creative about how I lived life.

Deep down I knew the things my body and mind and soul were so desperate to hear. After all that happened, I thought, *Why not use my voice to speak life into myself first?* If I couldn't fill my own love tank with edifying and life-giving words, how could I ever help anyone else?

All of us have our voice—think about statements and words you repeat to yourself regularly. We would never want to verbally diminish or deflate someone we love, so why would we talk to *ourselves* like that? How would your perspective change if you started voicing work-arounds to yourself rather than speaking out your limitations? If you started articulating the amazing things you are capable of *rather* than the things that might be challenging you, what might change?

Maybe you miss going to your favorite Pilates or yoga class. Why not encourage yourself to go on YouTube and find some easy moves you can do in bed or on a chair in the privacy of your bedroom? Even if you can only last two minutes the first time, look at it as two minutes of growth, moving you from where you were previously. There are even a variety of exercise videos online specifically for someone who is struggling with a chronic illness (you can even find some on my Instagram). Maybe like me you experience muscle pain when chopping vegetables or fruit or meat or when trying to prepare a meal. Is it possible to rework your budget to spring for the precut vegetables, fruit, or meat at the grocer so the work is done for you and you can expend the energy you do have elsewhere?

Fabulous Finds

Some Ways to Stay Active

Trying to keep active in some way but don't want to overdo it and cause a flare-up?

The following are some great search terms on You-Tube for exercises for those who are disabled or chronically ill:

- Chair yoga
- Bed Exercises
- Bed stretch exercises
- Exercise for disabled
- Chronically ill exercises

So much of change begins with our thoughts and how we perceive our situation. What are some work-arounds you might consider? And how can your faith give you that extra boost when you need it? We all have different areas of struggle, but I can share with you that anxiety and fear about what might happen with lupus and how my body seemed so unstable crippled me. Through refocusing my thoughts, through prayer and reading scripture—through paying attention to how God sent specific people with words of wisdom my way—I understood I had a choice. Either I could focus and fret on things that hadn't even happened yet or I could put my faith completely in God, no matter what was going to happen. But I knew I didn't have the energy or the brain capacity to do both.

When I felt like I was spiraling, I would reach for some of my favorite verses from scripture or quotes from role models about hope and resiliency that I had written down on index cards, keeping them nearby just in case I needed a reminder. These quotes ran the gamut and spoke to me about overcoming challenges, reminding me how strong I truly was and that even in the midst of disaster and fear, all was not lost—I could overcome this. Here are some of my favorites:

> The human capacity for burden is like bamboo—far more flexible than you'd ever believe at first glance.
>
> —Jodi Picoult

> But still, like air, I'll rise.
>
> —Maya Angelou

> Hope is a renewable option; if you run out of it at the end of the day, you get to start over in the morning.
>
> —Barbara Kingsolver

> Worrying is carrying tomorrow's load with today's strength—carrying two days at once. It is moving into tomorrow ahead of time. Worrying doesn't empty tomorrow of its sorrow, it empties today of its strength.
>
> —Corrie ten Boom

There is no force equal to a woman determined
to rise.

—W. E. B. Du Bois

Don't fret or worry. Instead of worrying, pray.
Let petitions and praises shape your worries into
prayers, letting God know your concerns. Before
you know it, a sense of God's wholeness, everything coming together for good, will come and
settle you down.

—Philippians 4:6 MSG

In time, I didn't even need the index cards anymore because
those verses and quotes were within me; I'd memorized them,
and they became my new normal. And soon, I was able to use
my voice, speak those lines of promise and hope to myself, and
talk myself out of those freak-out moments. With these words
that became part of me combined with prayers and silence and
listening and hope, my voice became stronger and stronger.

I became stronger. I became more resilient.

Through the process and the challenges, I realized that for me
and for many of us, the trauma or illness or injury we experience is
part of God's plan to encourage, support, educate, and speak life
into someone else's pain and trauma and challenge. I remember
the first time I had the thought, *What if God allowed everything
that just happened to me as part of a greater plan so that I could
help support others just taking that first step on their journey?*

To be honest, I was terrified at the thought. *Surely, God,
there must be someone way better equipped for that job than I
am!* When we allow ourselves to take on a disability or diagnosis
identity, we start to believe this straight-up lie that we no longer
have anything left to offer this world, that we are broken or not

valuable and therefore can't help anyone. But this lie can sink us deeper and deeper into the confines of our four walls, and pour water on the flames of our voice, and keep our God-given gift hidden from the world, hidden away from the trauma-suffering stranger in desperate need of our encouragement and support.

Am I, I asked myself, *going to let a lie or a false sickness identity stop me from using the voice God gave me? Or can I work with God's help to rebuild on a firm foundation, one that uses the voice and creative gifts I've been given and a message to share with others?* I began to consider the crucial building blocks used in this new construction.

I'll never forget one particular week in my life when I felt that sense of purpose and God's calling on my life. It was revealed to me in such a clear way, there was no denying it. My entire life I had believed I would work as a nurse in the medical field. All I saw was a lost opportunity. But God's vision was different. I had been writing voraciously since I returned home from the hospital. Soon I shared some things I'd written with some friends.

During this time, I was definitely feeling the itch to return to work somehow and start making money, but my options for work were severely limited. Growing up in a single-parent household with my mother and often being raised by my grandparents while she worked two jobs, working hard was in my blood. I actually really love to work. Now I found myself unable to work outside of the home; I had a mountain of hospital, doctor, medication, and medical bills; and I wasn't able to contribute financially to help my mom and grandmother. This all weighed heavily on me. Those index cards and a lot of prayer helped me not descend into my old thinking patterns that I was less than or a failure.

As I kept writing and praying, pleading with God to make a new sense of purpose clear to me, I prayed about knowing how stubborn I was and how I often questioned everything, and after months of asking for something to come about in my life to help me live out God's plan and help me contribute to society, I found the answer on Sunday night. I'll never forget that night, when I wrapped up one of my prayers: "God, please! I am begging you to show me what you want me to do. I have all the time in the world right now. Maybe it is something with all of this writing? Maybe something creative? Whatever it is, please give me something that will make me feel useful while also living out your purpose. I can't wait much longer—I feel like I am losing my mind trapped in this house. And by the way, speaking of this house, whatever I do I need to do from this house, since I am basically stuck here right now!" Ha, no pressure from me, God . . .

I was a little bossypants in those prayers. And patience still isn't my strongest suit (though it has gotten better, thank you, Jesus). Yet even with my impatient and overbearing prayers, God answered me. At first, I couldn't even believe it.

The following day after that prayer, I received an unexpected call from an editor at the local Christian newspaper in Fort Lauderdale. This was a major hundred-plus-page, beautiful, monthly, color newspaper reaching hundreds of thousands of people throughout Florida and beyond. The editor's name was Didi—someone I am honored to call my friend to this day—and through a friend of a friend, she had read something I had written and asked if I would volunteer to write an article as a test piece for future potential work. I could interview people by phone, she said, and send my pieces in by email.

I never had to set foot in the office.

I could do everything from home, from bed!

This was perfect.

This was God.

Would I? I held the phone away from my face and covered the mic area, looked up toward the heavens, and whispered, "Are you serious, God? You work fast! Thank you!" I wish I could tell you exactly how I responded to Didi, but in my excitement and eagerness, I was a blubbering mess. God had swung a door wide open. In my shock, excitement, and elation, I summoned all the energy I had in my body at the moment, leapt from my bed, and made a beeline for the kitchen, knowing there was a 99 percent chance my grandmother would be standing near the stove. My mom happened to be in the kitchen, too, at that very moment, and as the aroma of homemade sauce and basil and oregano filled the air, I took a deep breath and then the words fell from my lips so quickly they could barely understand me. Grandma handed me a bowl of sauce and a chunk of fresh, warm bread and said, "Sit, sit," motioning me to the table. "Now tell us again this good news . . . a little slower!" She laughed. As I swirled and soaked the bread in the warm, meaty sauce, I shared with them how God had literally answered my prayer overnight, and things were starting to become clear.

This one test piece turned into a voluntary journalism gig, which eventually led to a paid position as a staff writer at the newspaper and then an assistant editor position. This unexpected break into the world of media and journalism would eventually lead me to write for major media outlets—including Gannett, *U.S. News*, *Al Jazeera*, and Healthline, among others—and host numerous online video interviews.

But God knew my writing was going to start with that Christian newspaper. It was there I would hone my craft while also having the opportunity to interview incredible people doing extraordinary things inspired by their faith. It also helped build my faith during these crucial, vulnerable, challenging years. My life plan had crumbled, and I had no idea how to pick up the pieces—but God's plan? God's plan was perfect.

But Monday's blessing wasn't the only prayer God answered that week. I remember floating through the week, finally being able to put a physical feeling to the oft-used phrase of "being on cloud 9." Elation from the opportunity combined with support from my family and friends, alongside a growing feeling of worthiness and empowerment, propelled me into even longer and deeper prayer. If God was opening this door to writing, I wanted these words to matter, to be life changing.

And then that Friday night, I had an incredibly vivid dream.

God speaks differently to everyone, I know. But God often speaks to me loud and clear in my dreams, to the point where it's like a plan of action I literally receive to download and follow. When I have these dreams and follow the plans, they meet with success. Every single time without fail. And that is exactly what happened on this night. The dream involved me creating a community—online—where people would find hope and encouragement if they too were diagnosed with lupus or any other chronic, incurable condition. This would be a place where anyone—no matter where in the world they were located—could reach out and speak freely and be loved on in their moment of need. This dream eventually led to a very basic website and blog that would grow to be known as LupusChick.

I didn't know where it would lead, but I knew its goals were clear from the beginning. From that dream, I knew this community had to be built on four pillars. Everything on it had to be:

- Encouraging.
- Motivating.
- Educational.
- Inspirational.

That simple, that clear. Period.

At the time, in the early 2000s, there were only a handful of websites and blogs you could find that discussed lupus. And if you did find the online resources, you were lucky if there was even a full page of information on the topic.

For some reason, God put the task of reaching out to others in my hands. And I happily accepted. I knew when I woke up that morning that after weeks and months and years of prayers about the new course for my life, and all the reading, all the study of immune issues and nutrition, and all the desperation and hope in prayer, God's timing brought everything together. "All right God," I said, "I have no idea what I am doing, but I am going to build it, and I am going to put it ultimately in your control. Let's do this!"

Now, I don't know you personally, I may not know your story or your pain (and I am sure you have had your share of pain), but there is one thing about you I know without a doubt: God has given you a unique voice and a distinctive purpose and can use whatever you are going through to refine and shape you into the person whose voice can share your message with the world.

Think of the seed analogy I mentioned at the beginning of this book. The seed life cycle has resonance for our journey with chronic illness. When we are diagnosed with a disease, we find ourselves in a really dark place, with all we have being like a small seed buried in the dirt. We are alone; we are surrounded by life's dirt shoveled on top of us. We try to push our way out, but we are stuck in the dark. But as with a seed, so much is happening during that dark, quiet, lonely time of all that is unknown.

Think of all the processes that occur to a tiny seed when it is placed in that dark, isolated environment. It is those processes it is undergoing that allow it to transform, bring forth growth, and begin to set down deep roots that will make it a strong, living plant. And with each little smidgen of growth, eventually the seedling pushes its way out of the dirt and into this extraordinary light and freedom and space, and it flourishes and bears fruit.

We're as various as the thousand distinctive seed varieties that produce different types of fruit in this world. We have unique fruit and purpose. Whether you love to write, speak to a crowd, act, paint, make art, lead, or teach a class, all of these are messages to be shared in a distinctive way, speaking life into the lives of others.

And whether you are mobile or immobile, bedbound or hospital bound, whatever gift God gave you, God will also make a way for it to unfold. God knows the exact voice you have and the timing and platform for how your story needs to be shared. When we say yes to God and to our lives—and our new life challenges—we can speak encouragement and hope into the lives of those who are scared or lonely or have lost hope for their lives given their circumstances.

The first thing we are called to do to bring the plan to fruition is to get out of our own way—to move past the fears, shame, or embarrassment we may feel and any worry and anxiety. When we take that first step forward in sharing our struggles openly and being transparent with the world, that seed begins to push into the light. And we are able to share our stories in our special way, as we have gifts and use those gifts. That might mean sharing your story in a private forum, perhaps over a delicious meal with a new friend who is struggling or scared. Or maybe God's journey for you will lead to a TED Talk stage, where millions will eventually hear your message. Each setting holds the same level of importance because each setting is the platform God is giving *you* to share a message that cannot be found through anyone else on the planet.

Your story is one of a kind.

Your journey through that dark, cold, lonely environment and how you pushed through and thrived? No one else can tell *that* exact story because it is uniquely yours.

And you're going to tell that story not from the viewpoint of a sick you, or a broken you, or a damaged you—or maybe all of those—but from a powerful you, a hopeful you, a you that you have co-conspired with God to create!

So whether God's path for you is to create a personal blog about how the chronic illness you have affects intimacy and dating, or whether it's a path leading you to travel around the world filming a documentary about some aspect of your struggle, or whether you find yourself making art or clothing that supports and encourages other people who are at the beginning of their diagnosis journey, whatever it is, don't hide it from this world.

Don't let an illness make you hesitate and question yourself, and don't deny yourself that satisfaction of seeing God's work in and through you. God put so much into creating something in you to come to fruition. Use that God-given voice. Let it speak out of you into the lives of others the way God spoke it into you when creating you.

Easy Chickpea Pasta Salad

Prep Time: 10 minutes
Cook Time: 10–15 minutes
Yield: 4 servings

Looking for a pasta dish that isn't heavy? This summery version is not only light but very versatile. I use chickpea pasta, but depending on your preference, you can also use rice, lentil, or wheat pasta. The best part of this recipe, which you don't want to skip, is my version of my grandmother's tangy vinegar dressing. It is a tastebud extravaganza that combines sweetness with tangy with loads of flavor. Fresh garlic mixed with honey, lemon, and other healthy ingredients round out this easy dish. The dressing recipe is a key component to this dish, but since it is intense, I would recommend you pour only half of the finished product on the pasta dish, stir, and taste. If you want more flavor, use a little more. I typically use about half of the dressing recipe on the pasta (and save the rest as dip for warm bread with butter). Enjoy!

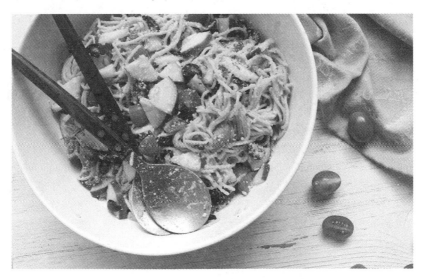

Pasta

12 oz chickpea spaghetti (I prefer the Explore Cuisine brand)
1 cucumber, diced or cut into boat rounds
1 cup small cherry tomatoes, quartered
1 can medium or large black (or Kalamata) olives, each sliced in half
   or quartered
½ cup grated parmigiano reggiano cheese or grated cheese
   substitute, optional

Grandma Rosie's Tangy Homemade Italian Dressing

½ cup olive oil
½ cup apple cider vinegar
1 large clove of fresh garlic, pressed
1 juice of a medium lemon
1½ teaspoons honey
½ teaspoon pink Himalayan salt
½ teaspoon black pepper
1 teaspoon dried basil
1 teaspoon dried oregano

Prepare your mise en place. I generally start by making the dressing. Combine olive oil, apple cider vinegar, lemon, honey, fresh garlic, salt, pepper, and spices. Mix very well and store in a container with a tight lid.

Next, boil water in a large pot and prepare chickpea pasta according to instructions on the package. When fully cooked, drain and rinse quickly with cold water.

Place the pasta in a large bowl and add cucumbers, tomatoes, olives, parmigiano reggiano cheese, and half of the dressing. Mix very well. Taste and add more dressing if you want. Top with extra cheese if desired and enjoy!

NINE

A Fortress Made of True Friends

*Friendship is born at that moment when
one person says to another: "What! You
too? I thought I was the only one."*
—C. S. Lewis

Whether someone is chronically ill or not, the ever-changing cycle of relationships—both platonic and intimate—is something we all encounter. As a myriad of internal and external changes take place once a diagnosis occurs, it's important to support our relationships and understand how illness can affect them or how they affect our illness.

Healthy relationships are essential to well-being, and this is especially true when we are suffering from an illness. Those we keep closest to us influence our work. The biblical book of Ecclesiastes tells us that two are better than one, so if one falls down, there is another to help them up. In other places in scripture, relationships, we're told, help us "sharpen" one another.

And treating each other kindly, as we'd want to be treated, is something we're called to live out in our relationships. These challenging, supporting, kind friendships are ones we crave and are taught to aim for.

The Hebrew Bible also cautions us about what happens when we are part of or support harmful relationships—they are not only harmful to others but take us off course. While in the best of times we might know which relationships nurture us, sometimes chronic illness can make the waters of relationships murky, confusing, and even painful. The truth is, some of the most unkind things we may hear in relation to our illness might come from those closest to us. And those people we thought for sure would help us up when we fall? Well, they might not stick around at all.

So what do the platonic and romantic relationships in our life have to do with our health and a new diagnosis? Everything. Because our mental and physical states are so intimately connected, we need to take inventory of the people who are speaking into our life. And we need to discern if the words spoken and the actions taken toward us are life-giving or life-taking. Chronic illness is going to teach us a lot about ourselves—such as the limits of our physical and mental strength, how faith shapes us, how we understand our mindset, our endurance, our flexibility, and how patient we are in meeting challenging situations. It's also going to tell us a lot about the relationships we have with our partners, family members, friends, acquaintances . . . and believe it or not, even strangers.

Here is something you should know about chronic illness.

It is going to rearrange your relationships.

Some of this rearrangement may be painful, but in the long run, you'll come to recognize it is also necessary. When you become chronically ill and cannot do all of the things you once did, or make every event, or help out with every family activity, or meet up with your friends every weekend, or go hit up happy hour or a restaurant with your buddies after work, the harsh reality is that the people you thought you knew and could rely on, you'll realize you didn't know so well.

On the other hand, some people will surprise you.

You'll find they are willing to educate themselves and want to understand more about your diagnosis and how it is restructuring your life. These are the people whose friendships or relationships with you aren't superficial but go deep. Even though you may not be able to meet them out somewhere, or help them at an event or activity, or necessarily "do" anything for them during this season of your life, they are willing to come to you, even if it is just to sit on your bed and talk, watch Netflix, bring you food, or wipe your tears when you are a complete disaster.

Thank God for these people.

These are the people who, even though they may not completely understand why you aren't "getting better" or why you may deal with limitations for a long time, aren't going to drop you like a hot potato when your illness places a massive speed bump dead center in the journey of your friendship.

Others, you'll discover, eventually move forward with their lives without you because you and your chronic illness no longer work for their needs. Stating it like that sounds harsh. And it is. For those left by those they thought were friends, it may also seem extremely selfish. But I prefer to look at it differently. I see it as God weeding out the people who don't need to be in our immediate circle. These are the types of relationships— whether platonic or intimate—that make you scratch your head and think, *Wow, I really thought our relationship was stronger than this.* Sometimes we're completely caught off guard when these relationships begin to crumble.

Your relationship can deteriorate when the other person either is unable to understand your illness or doesn't fully comprehend or *even believe* that you are not well and that you're no longer able to play the same role you once did in the relationship. For whatever reason, they cannot or will not adjust. The breakdown of these relationships can hurt you deep within your soul. And sometimes, heartbreaking words may be spoken to you that rattle you and are held in your memory bank for years to come. Here are some of the phrases I've heard that are etched deep in my mind:

"You're still sick?"
"So you're going to *cancel again*?"
"I feel like you aren't trying hard enough to get better!"

Fabulous Finds

The 10 LupusChick Elements of True Friendship

- support
- reliability
- confidentiality
- deep listening
- nonjudgmental presence
- trust
- interdependence
- care
- responsiveness
- mutuality

"You just want attention!"

"You look great—are you sure you're not faking it?"

"I just can't be with someone who is sick all the time."

How these words sting! And they make us want to cry out in response:

I'm chronically ill, which means it is part of my life every single day. I never get a break or a day off.

I hate the fact that I have to cancel—yes, again—but the best thing I can do for my body right now is rest.

I'm battling this every single day and using every ounce of energy just to keep up with the bare minimum of survival!

This isn't what I would want attention for! I had goals and dreams, and illness wasn't any part of what I hoped to gain attention for.

I can't fake a stroke, or blood clot, or brain aneurysm, or (insert other health crisis here)!

Thank you for telling me now, because one day God will bless me with someone who sees my worth far beyond this illness and will love me the way God loves me.

And as if those stinging remarks aren't hurtful enough when friends speak them to us, sometimes we'll hear those comments from our own family members. Now, those can cut really deep. Some of the most damaging and traumatizing comments I heard after my diagnosis came from my own family. From people I thought would rally around me and want to help me.

For some reason, these people were unable to understand how someone could be sick for more than a few days, or how someone who used to run around all over the place and work all hours of the night could no longer even bathe herself. For me, I understood these comments were made by family members who had never dealt with any serious or chronic illnesses personally and therefore didn't have firsthand knowledge or understanding of how a chronic illness can change your entire life and force you to adapt to a new normal. Sometimes responses like that indicate they are unsure of how to adapt alongside you, or perhaps they aren't ready to adapt, and their own frustration and ignorance and fear fall out of their mouths in painful words, stinging the second they are spoken.

When we are first met with shocking and hurtful reactions from friends and family, we may try to explain our illness to them until we are blue in the face—in some cases we try dozens of times to explain. Or we might push ourselves physically to attend an event or do a chore because we want to please them, or be accepted, or seem like "our old self," even if just for a moment. No one wants to feel different, or blacklisted, or shunned, but that is exactly what these kinds of ignorant comments do. They negatively affect our physical *and* mental health. This is not okay, and this is not what God wants for us. If friendship is caring for and loving one another as we love ourselves, how does it work that friendship can be found in trivializing or invalidating someone's illness experience?

The relationship losses I experienced in those first few years when I was almost completely hospital and home bound taught me some tough life lessons. In addition to recovering from my injuries, it took doctors a long time to get a good diagnosis for and treatment handle on the lupus and other autoimmune issues I was experiencing. I was clocking in dozens of hospital admissions annually. When I wasn't in the hospital, I was typically at home recovering (because we all know you get *zero* rest in the hospital). Not only did I have to mentally reconcile losing my nursing career, and my independence, and much of my finances (which went to medical bills), but I was also hit with the loss of relationships.

At first, it seemed like my friends held on, but as time went by, more and more fell to the wayside. I tried as best as I could to keep in contact during the times I had enough energy to carry on a conversation. I noticed the first group of friends to go were those who were in nursing school with me. I thought we were a tight bunch—we were in the program together for several years, taking each class together, studying together, staying late after school to prepare for tests, and doing our rotations together. But between their hectic schedules of school and rotation rounds and the fact that we were never together physically anymore, those friendships quickly dissolved. Soon, I noticed friendships I had made through work (I was a bartender during college) and even some of my long-term platonic relationships just couldn't handle the strain of my illness. I was too sick to put in any more effort, and I couldn't fault them for living their lives.

Many times I would stare outside a hospital window and feel like life was happening all around me and I wasn't a part of any of it. But I also was aware that God blessed me with a core group of loving friends who stepped up in the years following my diagnosis. They were the ones who helped prevent me from falling deep into despair from loneliness. They were the faithful friends who never made me feel left out. The health and maturity of these relationships were even deepened by their willingness to forge ahead and love on me despite the obstacles around and ahead of us.

When we are handed a diagnosis, we all need support, encouragement, love, hope, and assurance that people are walking this journey with us. And it will surprise you who, in the long run, sticks by your side and offers this beautiful gift of friendship.

Equally surprising will be the discovery of those who have moved away from you in this season of your life.

Over the years, I've had a tight circle of people who have stuck with me. And at this point in our lives, I believe there isn't anything that can be thrown at us that would cause us to separate. My friend Alan would drive me to the hospital and then bring every board game known to man in order to help distract me from the long hospital days that seemed to melt into one another. Ever the prankster, he would play jokes on the nurses and always get us involved in some type of ridiculous shenanigans, and we would literally laugh until we were crying. I may not remember exactly what we were laughing about back then, but I will always remember those deep belly laughs where we would both be short of breath and our sides would hurt.

My best friend, Karla, has basically become an extension of my body over the years. Our early morning coffee conversations, and an additional five or six phone or video calls per day, help

Fabulous Finds

What Friendship Means

Home. "When I look at you, I can feel it. I look at you and I'm home." —Dory, *Finding Nemo*

Multiplication of all that is good. "True friendship multiplies the good in life and divides its evils." —Baltasar Gracián

Life support. "Some people arrive and make such a beautiful impact on your life, you can barely remember what life was like without them." —Anna Grace Taylor

us stay intimately connected even in the seasons when I cannot physically leave my bed. Not only has she acted as a living example of someone with a profound faith, but she has been there for me daily—through all kinds of situations and emotions and drama—and loved me unconditionally every step of the way. God knew I needed a sassy, spunky sidekick who could finish my sentences and match my strange sense of humor, and I have no doubt God planned for our lives to collide many years ago. And my pals Cici, Tony, and Petagaye (whom I have been close to since my teenage years), are my no-nonsense, shoot-it-to-you-straight, love-you-every-step-of-the-way besties. These are the ones you can call any hour of the day or night and share your deepest secrets, thoughts, and fears with and know there won't be any judgment—just love. We all need friends like these.

Most surprising to me in this journey of chronic illness and friendships were the friends I would make *after* I was diagnosed. I heard it said once that chronic illness has the power to turn friends into strangers and strangers into friends, and I don't think there is any better description than that.

When LupusChick began to take off, people began engaging with me and one another, and I started attending illness support groups and advocating for lupus at certain events. As a result, I was suddenly introduced to a tribe that I didn't know ever existed and didn't know how desperately I needed! I felt like I had entered into a secret dimension where people were dealing with the same struggles I faced daily, understood my greatest illness-related fears and concerns, and didn't judge me if I didn't respond for a few days, or couldn't make it to an event, or had to take a time out, or disappeared into the bathroom for two hours. And while they didn't necessarily verbalize it, there was an understanding that poured out from these men and women that said, "You are safe here. You're one of us." And I finally felt free, like I could be myself—my new self, lupus and all—and it was okay.

Relationships are given to us for mutual support and encouragement and love. In the book of Genesis, God said it's not good for humankind to be alone. When the Creator fashioned the world, one of the greatest creative acts was the creation of companions.

Speaking of companions, some relationships may come about in ways that we never expected. We may not meet a new friend at school or at our job during this season of our life, but we may just find that unexpected person we click with on an online medical forum, or through a Facebook post conversation, or sitting across from us at an in-person support group or in the same doctor's waiting room. They may be the roommate in our hospital room, or someone we find inspirational in our Instagram or TikTok feed, or a friend of a friend.

They are out there. It's up to us to have faith and to believe that while some of our friendships or relationships may feel like they have come to an end or have been strained, God—who created us for relationship with each other and with the Divine—isn't going to let us travel this journey alone.

And while some of us may be yearning for a special platonic friendship with someone experiencing a situation similar to ours, others may be looking for something deeper, something romantic. But with the challenges just our friendships alone can present, the thought of trying to *date* with a chronic illness can almost paralyze us. On one hand, we want love and companionship, and on the other, we ask ourselves, How can I bring someone else into this whirlwind when I feel like some days I am barely hanging on myself?

When I first contemplated dating a while after I was diagnosed, I successfully talked myself out of it in about thirty seconds. What if they can't handle that I get sick a lot or that I may have to cancel dates with them at the last minute? Who is going to want to sit with me at the hospital when they could be out doing something they enjoy? How can I be a wife, and have children, and take care of my spouse if I can barely bathe and feed myself some days? What happens when I get physical side effects from the medicine I take and I begin to look different—would someone still like me? *No, no, no. Surely, no one is going to want to deal with all of this and more when there are so many healthy, available people out there*, I thought to myself.

And even though I adore God, and knew the person I was created to be, and shared in a sense of purpose with God, I was still somehow unable to conclude that I was worthy to be with anyone else, because my illness made me feel less than. I minimized all that God made me, and for a long time, I believed the lie that no one could truly love me in this new package I came in. For years I self-sabotaged potential relationships anytime someone showed interest. And finally I resigned to the fact that I was going to focus solely on my work and the purpose God had for me, because I was likely meant to be alone forever.

But sure enough, God had other plans.

During a rare night of energy, I walked into a karaoke event near my house and locked eyes with the most beautiful man I had ever met. Tall, with blonde hair, blue eyes, and a perfect smile, he looked like a cast member from *Baywatch*. His name was Mickey, but I'd later come to find out that some of his friends had nicknamed him "Baywatch"! All he was missing was that comic-book-like glint and sparkle when he flashed his pearly whites. And he loved Jesus to boot. And despite lupus, and the fact that I would disappear for weeks on end when my health got rocky and completely dodge him, and my hundreds of attempts to push him away to date someone "healthy," that tender spirited, easygoing, God-loving, rare unicorn of a man saw something extraordinary in me—and never gave up on us.

And despite all of my resistance and second-guessing about whether he was going to have a moment of clarity at any second and run for the hills, we fell deeply in love with one another and began riding out the roller coaster life that is chronic illness together, with a shared hope in God to guide us.

That isn't to say it has been a bed of roses since the moment our eyes first locked on to each other. Chronic illness can bring some bizarre and stressful experiences to a romantic relationship. But when two people have a commitment to each other, these experiences can also bring them closer as they work through anything that might be thrown their way—together.

Both God and Mickey are responsible for teaching me truths about myself that I couldn't see on my own and that I am worthy and deserving of love just as I am. Those of us who have chronic illness often sell ourselves short, we compare ourselves to healthy people (who, by the way, have their own issues!), and we come up with every reason or excuse for why no one would want to intentionally deal with the hills and valleys of our illness. Sometimes we even try to convince ourselves that there is no way even *God* could love us in our present condition. But why do we try to talk ourselves out of the love that God wants to bring into our life?

Some say that illness will push people away from deeper connections with you. Don't believe it. God offers faithful friendship with different timing, and that allows us to recognize our worth. That allows us to understand that this diagnosis is just a small fraction of who we are. When someone can see that your struggles and pain have refined you rather than defined you and have brought about incredible growth rather than impeded growth, thank God for that soul—whether it is a romantic partner or a best friend. Because when you find that, you have found your person. And that, my friend, is a beautiful, God-given thing.

Easy Vegetarian Moroccan Chickpea Stew

Prep Time: 25 minutes
Cook Time: 4.5–5 hours on high
Method: Stovetop and slow cooker
Yield: 6 servings

This is one of my all-time favorite shared meals. Typically, I have a slow cooker of it brewing every weekend, and I make it any time a friend or family member comes into town. I prefer to serve mine over jasmine rice, but you can also serve it over quinoa, orzo, or brown rice. You can also top it with avocado or Greek yogurt. If you aren't a fan of chickpeas, you could swap them out for cannellini beans. This stew is packed with fiber, protein, and nutrients, plus it is warming and comforting on a chilly fall or winter day. My favorite part? If I am not feeling great or my energy is low, the majority of the work is done by the slow cooker (which gives me plenty of time to rest!).

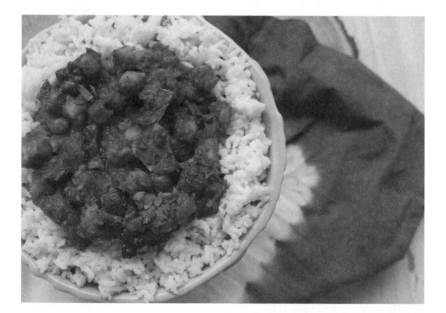

· · · · · · · · · · · · · · **INGREDIENTS** · · · · · · · · · · · · · · ·

1–2 tablespoons olive oil
1 sweet Vidalia onion, chopped
6 cloves garlic, pressed or minced (or 6 teaspoons minced jar garlic)
2 cans chickpeas, drained and rinsed
2 cups vegetable broth
One 6-ounce can of tomato paste
One 14.5-ounce can petite diced tomatoes
2 medium sweet potatoes, skin removed, cubed
2 zucchini, skin on, cubed
1 teaspoon cinnamon
1 teaspoon cumin
2 teaspoons garam masala
½ teaspoon turmeric
½ teaspoon ginger powder
Dash or two of cayenne or chili pepper
3 tablespoons maple syrup
Himalayan or sea salt and pepper (season as you like)
10 pitted dates, chopped and set aside

Optional
Rice
Orzo
Quinoa
Avocado
Greek yogurt
Fresh basil or cilantro to garnish

Add olive oil to a pan and heat on medium-high heat. Add onion, stir to combine with oil, and cook for 3–4 minutes. Next, add garlic and cook for 1–2 minutes. Transfer mixture to your slow cooker. Add all ingredients except for the dates. Stir well. Cover and secure slow cooker, turn on high, and cook for 4 hours (stirring occasionally during this time). At the 4-hour mark, add chopped dates to slow cooker and stir. Cover and cook for another 30–60 minutes, until the sweet potatoes are soft. Serve alone or over rice, orzo, or quinoa. Top with avocado or Greek yogurt, if you like.

TEN

Flares, Frankfurters, and Other Catastrophes

The act of living is different all through. Her
absence is like the sky, spread all over everything.
—C. S. Lewis

Grief is like living two lives—one where you pretend
that everything is alright, and the other
where your heart silently screams in pain.
—Unknown

Life can often be full of wonder, and joy, and unforgettable moments, but if we are being realistic, we'll also acknowledge that life can be messy, unpredictable, and stressful. Just when we think we have everything together and organized and are ready to tie off that shiny red bow to showcase how neatly packaged our mess is, life gets creative and throws us some real humdingers. Add to this challenge that autoimmune disease and chronic illness flares are often triggered by stress, and it doesn't take a rocket scientist to see that combo isn't good.

Dealing with stressors—both internal and external—and the occasional crisis that happens to all of us at some time or another while we are still learning to live with and adjust to a diagnosis can be tricky. And it doesn't matter which autoimmune disease or chronic illness you have, or your personality, or how much you "have it together," or how resilient you are; there is an adjustment period for all of us.

At some point, we all come to recognize that stress—both good and bad stress—affects how our bodies respond. It influences a person's disease state—sometimes so much so that an unexpected period of stress or a major event can cause a flare-up that knocks us right off our feet and onto our butt.

In the first few years after I was diagnosed with lupus, I had very little awareness of the impact that stress had on my symptoms and how much it correlated with my flares. It turns out that alongside certain foods and lack of sleep, stress was one of my main flare triggers. Although I had begun journaling and tracked my sleep and nap periods, what I ate, what events were happening, medications and supplements I was taking, doctors' appointments, hospitalizations, my menstrual cycle, and more, I hadn't yet accumulated enough data to be able to review and see clear trends and connections between stress and the rising number of symptoms, such as fever, increased fatigue, mouth and nose sores, and rashes. And sometimes a flare would knock me down for days or weeks.

When one particular earth-shattering event occurred, I got an instant reality check. It was through this experience and my body's response that I would come to fully understand the result of the toxic combination of stress and autoimmune disease. After that point, I would focus on learning how to balance various areas of my life in order to keep the scales from tipping into dangerous territory.

When Mickey proposed to me in a quaint log cabin during a chilly fall evening on a trip to Gatlinburg, Tennessee, I was ecstatic. I had finally been healthy enough to travel for a few days away from home, and Mickey wanted to share the fall foliage and beauty that happens in the area during this season. We were drinking warm cinnamon-apple tea with honey, I was wrapped up in a fuzzy cardigan, and we were sprawled out on the floor, playing cards. Growing up playing cards weekly with my grandparents, aunts, uncles, and cousins on what I would call "coffee klatch" night (where the entire table was filled with desserts and coffee), I loved the fact that Mickey also enjoyed playing cards with me. During this particular game, I pulled a card from the options in his hand, and attached to the other side of the card was a stunning antique wedding ring. It was there, in this beautiful, peaceful, dim cabin where Mickey asked me to spend the rest of our days together. Shortly after, when the shock and excitement leveled off, I grabbed my phone to call Grandma and Mom to share the news.

When we arrived back home a few days later, I ran into my grandmother's house to show my family the beautiful ring and tell them all about our adventures. Even though I was over the moon to marry Mickey, my grandmother may have been even more excited than I was! From the first day she met Mickey, she adored him. He never really had the opportunity to be with his grandmother, so mine sort of became his adopted Italian nonna. They would talk for hours, he would take her to events like *Dancing with the Stars* when it came to our town (it was her favorite TV show aside from *Days of Our Lives*), and she loved the fact that she had one more person to feed on a regular basis (and Mickey can really eat!).

The two of them would have their own version of Grandma/soon-to-be-son-in-law date nights sometimes when I was in a flare and sleeping it off in my bedroom. I would often wake from a nap in the early evening to find them relaxing in the living room, chowing down on one of my grandmother's favorite vices—Costco hot dogs.

Don't even get me started . . .

This is a woman who could literally cook anything anyone wanted, but the kitchen would come to an immediate close when Mickey would show up at the door with a tray of Costco hot dogs, enough sauerkraut to feed a small village, mustard, and a movie.

Though my grandma was a little wisp of a thing, we used to liken her to a bull. The woman never got sick . . . despite her continuous consumption of frankfurter ingredients. In fact, I can only remember her being sick one time when I was in my early twenties. She was hospitalized after having a mild heart attack. She and my mom both quit smoking cold turkey that very day. Even though Grandma had been smoking for more than fifty years at that point and knew it wasn't going to be easy to quit, that rare stint in the hospital scared her enough that the motivation to not die outweighed whatever satisfaction she got from her cigarettes.

I knew her as a strong and resilient woman most of my life, so about a year after Mickey proposed and we were on our honeymoon, I was completely thrown off guard when my mom called to tell us that Grandma had been rushed to the hospital. At ninety-two years old, Grandma's prognosis of pneumonia, extremely high blood pressure, and a collapsed lung wasn't a good one.

It was almost midnight when I got off the phone with my mother, and I sat on the edge of the bed in our hotel room. A sudden tightness in my chest appeared, the same one I felt in the hospital so many years ago. I prayed, but I knew an anxiety attack had already started, and I would need to ride it out. After twenty minutes or so passed—minutes filled with more prayers and my go-to pursed-lip breathing practice for such moments—it subsided. I sprang up from the bed. "We have to leave this hotel as soon as possible," I said. As we were only a four-hour drive from home, Mickey and I decided to pack up right then and head for the hospital. The drive back home was a complete blur; besides a few intense prayers for healing and for the chance to see my grandmother one more time, we drove in complete silence.

When we finally arrived at the hospital, Mickey dropped me off at an entrance, and I couldn't get up to her room fast enough. I slowed my pace as I entered her room, as it was very early in the morning, and I stood there for several minutes just staring at her, watching her breathe. Her face was sunken in, and her body exhibited an unfamiliar air of frailty and exhaustion. My eyes traveled along the maze of IV lines and wires attached to monitors, machines, and her body. She stirred and slowly opened her eyes, and in that moment, I rushed over to the bed. I needed to hold her and be as close as possible to her, so I curled up alongside my grandmother right there in the hospital bed and told her over and over again how much she was adored and loved and that she would be all right.

Over the next few days, Mickey, my mother, and I basically lived at the hospital, rotating visitation shifts. Grandma and I had many wonderful conversations during this time, and we watched *Days of Our Lives* every single day. I read to her when she felt too tired, helped her with her dollar-store crossword puzzles, brushed her hair, gently massaged her feet, and fed her chocolate pudding and chicken soup in the rare moments her appetite returned. All kinds of plans were made about the things she and Mickey and I were going to do when she was released from the hospital.

With every fiber of my being, I believed she was coming home.

There was no doubt in my mind that there would be family meals cooked together in Mickey's and my new home and even more movie and Costco hot dog nights.

And then one morning, most likely from the stress of the wedding, traveling for the honeymoon, the sudden decline in my grandmother's health, and lack of sleep, I woke up with a wicked fever, a body rash, and such intense fatigue that I could barely bring myself to the bathroom, let alone dress and get over to the hospital. Throughout that day, when I would wake from yet another nap, I would try once again to get ready and fail every single time. So Mickey and I decided he would take my place that evening and go visit Grandma for a few hours, and I would then return in the morning. I felt terrible for not being at the hospital, but knowing how much she enjoyed time with Mickey, there was a peace about staying back just this one day and letting them have time together.

That night, I fell into a deep, uninterrupted sleep, my body soaking in every minute of rest it was given. When I finally rolled over at around 8:15 the next morning, seventeen missed calls were displayed on my phone's home screen. Instantly my heartbeat shifted and my body went into high alert.

There was no need to listen to the dozen-plus voice mails stored in my phone; I already knew in my heart what the messages were going to say. My hands began shaking uncontrollably as I scrolled through my phone to find the last call from my mother. I reached over to wake Mickey, raising my voice: "Mickey, get up. Get up, now. Something's wrong. We have to go, come on." I dialed my mom, and before I could even ask what happened, she shared, "She's gone, Marisa. She died very early this morning."

I hung up the phone, and in a stunned, robotic demeanor, I pulled the covers back over me, made my body small, and tucked myself deep into Mickey's arms. There were a few minutes of silence before deep, guttural cries poured from my body along with waves of tears. A sudden and tremendous guilt washed over me, reminding me of the one night, the one stupid night I couldn't get myself there would have been the last opportunity to see her, hold her, and tell her for the millionth time how much I loved her.

Mickey drove me to the hospital, where my grandmother had been moved to a different room—large and sterile—where she was lying on an oversized metal slab with a thin, rough fabric sheet covering her body. I was heartbroken, and angry, and confused by her being relocated to such a cold and heartless environment that seemed to strip her or any human being that wound up here of their dignity. To the hospital employees, she was just another patient who passed, but for me, she was my life: my grandmother and mother and best friend and mentor and supporter and teacher and role model all rolled into one tiny, strong body. I held my grandmother for a long time, running my hands through her hair, speaking softly into her ear, and using every ounce of energy not to break down in the moment. When it was time for them to take her body, I asked the nurse for a scissor and a piece of tape and cut a large lock of her wavy, thick, now silvery-auburn hair and tucked it into my pocket.

Years prior, before the accident, I had struggled with the death of my grandfather. But even that experience in no way prepared me for the depth of this loss. Though I believed in my heart that my grandmother was beginning her new journey in heaven, everything here on earth suddenly felt incomplete and as though it was moving in slow motion. I was also experiencing my first monumental loss as someone living with a chronic illness that wasn't well controlled. I wasn't prepared for a heartbreak alongside my wide variety of physical symptoms. This was a challenge to navigate: not only dealing with the loss of someone I loved but also figuring out how to walk the fine line between allowing myself to grieve and somehow controlling the amount of physical and emotional pressure grief put on my body.

Over the following weeks, it was as if all of my common sense and nuggets of wisdom I had learned about how to better care for myself went out the window. During a hazy, rare trip out of the house to the grocery store, I strolled the aisles in a fog, unsure of what I was looking for. I passed by my grandmother's favorite Stella Doro Swiss Fudge cookies and had a massive anxiety attack in the aisle. Abandoning my cart, I ran to my car right then and there. After that incident, what I can only describe as a deep situational depression put me in bed for over three weeks straight. While some people turn to food or other feel-good vices during challenging seasons, I tend to lean in the opposite direction, losing my appetite completely. In fact, I don't remember eating for most of this three-week period. My only strong recollection from this time is waking from my bed, walking into my bathroom and drinking from the faucet, and returning right back to sleep. For me, this grief was imposing, and it demanded to be felt. I tried my hardest to pray during this time for God's peace and strength, but sorrow seemed to be winning out every single time.

By week three of little food and complete heartbreak, I felt as though I had gone backward years in terms of both my physical health and the closeness I felt with God. I was covered in rashes, I had a consistent fever for weeks and a mouth full of sores, my hair began falling out, and my heart felt "funny." With barely enough energy to stand, I forced myself downstairs knowing if I didn't eat soon, there would likely be a hospital trip in *my* near future.

Navigating the staircase was a slow and exhausting process, my legs shaky and weak from weeks lying in bed. As I neared the bottom of the staircase, I paused three stairs up from the first-floor landing and stared at the kitchen directly in front of me. I felt complete numbness as I scanned the appliances and food items scattered along the countertop. It hit me: *I will never cook in my brand-new kitchen with my grandmother. In fact, I will never cook with her again. Period.* Unexpectedly, feelings of anger and resentment crept in. The thought of setting foot in that kitchen suddenly disgusted me. I could feel my blood pressure rising. I was suddenly so mad, and I didn't understand why. I felt mad at God and even angrier at my grandmother for leaving me here without her. It was selfish and irrational, but I felt it with every fiber of my being. But underneath it all, I was mostly angry at myself and my failing body for being unable to be there that night. That very last night.

Memories flooded my brain as I stood there, each memory a remembrance of my grandmother and me cooking up something magical. Whether it was passing each other spices, taking a taste from the wooden spoon, or laughing about something silly while we cooked, the memories completely shattered my heart, knowing "one more time" was now an impossibility. My grandmother believed in her heart that one could heal any ailment with food, and I know in a time of heartache and sorrow and grief, she would have been the first person to feed me something soul warming, like lemony chicken soup and our house staple, pastina. But I couldn't step past that third step, let alone into the kitchen, to get my hands on the very items I knew my body and my heart were in desperate need of. In this moment, I felt like I, too, no longer wanted to or needed to be here.

Instead, I crawled into a ball right there. As my body tucked into itself, I realized I felt so very far away from God. Overwhelmed with loss, I was aware I hadn't really learned how to lean on God in this type of situation. Right there on that staircase, I prayed for strength to deal with the loss. I prayed for peace in knowing that I would see my grandmother again one day and that this was not the finite end it now felt like.

Maybe it sounds silly, but on that step, I also prayed for an appetite and for these feelings of disgust and disdain and anger that I felt about food and being in the kitchen to go away. The kitchen had always been this magical place that was both the birthplace and the guardian of a lifetime of unreplaceable memories. I knew the last thing my grandmother would want was for this event to be the reason I never set foot in a kitchen again.

And as I maneuvered my feeble body from that step, I prayed for God's presence to flood the situation. Despite being surrounded by so many family and friends, I felt so completely alone without my grandmother. But I knew I would need to force myself to eat and begin physically nourishing my fragile body that was also so utterly depleted and malnourished in the spiritual sense.

What I was *actually* hungry for had nothing to do with food but everything to do with God. I poured my heart out to God in a whisper that afternoon right there on the third step, my voice weak from exhaustion. Soon after, my face itchy from being buried deep in the rough, wiry fibers of the carpet, I dreamt of my grandmother smiling, the lines etched into her face that made her the beautiful woman she was. I dreamt of the last time I held her hands at the hospital, my young, soft fingers interwoven with hers that carried a lifetime of experience and wisdom. And when I awoke, I cried myself back to sleep.

Warm Golden Milk

Prep/Cook Time: 10 minutes
Method: Stovetop
Yield: 1 serving

Maybe you can't, like my grandmother believed, heal *every* ailment with food or spices, but there's something about golden milk that gets very close. It's one of my favorite ways to consume turmeric/curcumin—a favorite ingredient in immune-challenged communities. This recipe contains coconut oil and black pepper to help your body better absorb the incredible rewards of this spice. (Black pepper contains piperine, which can help increase turmeric/curcumin absorption by 2,000 percent!)

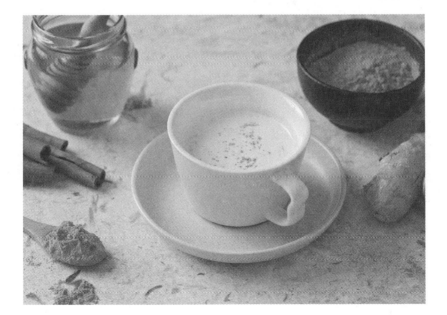

· · · · · · · · · · · · · · · **INGREDIENTS** · · · · · · · · · · · · · · ·

Turmeric Paste
½ cup filtered water
½ teaspoon ground black pepper
¼ cup organic turmeric powder

Before making the golden milk recipe, first make the tumeric paste. Place all ingredients into a small saucepan and heat on medium, constantly stirring until the mixture forms a thick paste. This should take about 5 minutes. You can store the paste in a glass jar in the refrigerator for up to 10 days.

Golden Milk
½–1 teaspoon of your turmeric paste
1 cup coconut milk (or other milk alternative)
½ teaspoon organic coconut oil
¼ teaspoon ground cinnamon
⅛ teaspoon ground cardamom
1 teaspoon raw honey or pure maple syrup to sweeten
Nutmeg, optional

Heat your milk alternative, cinnamon, and cardamom in a small saucepan on medium heat, stirring frequently. Whisk in the turmeric paste, honey, and coconut oil and heat until steaming; do not boil. Strain off cardamom and cinnamon, and serve immediately. You can add extra raw honey or nutmeg for additional taste if you want the milk sweeter.

ELEVEN

The Heat of the Fire

*The Wilderness holds answers to more
questions than we have yet learned to ask.*
— Nancy Newhall

*The wilderness is an untamed, unpredictable
place of solitude and searching. It is a place
as dangerous as it is breathtaking, a place as
sought after as it is feared. But it turns out to be
the place of true belonging, and it's the bravest
and most sacred place you will ever stand.*
— Brené Brown

After the loss of my grandmother, I reviewed the many lessons I learned. But one stood out in particular: anyone—like me—with a chronic illness has to be extra vigilant with their health and well-being in the middle of dealing with loss, grief, or other life-altering events. When we're caught off guard and not properly prepared, these events can bring an already struggling body to a place of complete depletion and devastation. It becomes another life-altering event that is also difficult to rebound from.

That spiral that led to the come-back-to-Jesus moment on the staircase would be my worst lupus flare to date. In a matter of months, I had shifted from being a strong version of myself (i.e., the strongest since my diagnosis) to being completely broken physically and emotionally, suffering ministrokes, a blood clot, and brain aneurysm and being hospitalized twelve times within the following months, eventually leading to chemotherapy.

The combination of grieving my grandmother, a move, a budding journalism career, and a new marriage overwhelmed my brain and my body. While I was telling those around me that the exponential impact was too much on me, good-intentioned friends, family members, and church acquaintances told me, "God never gives you more than you can handle." Every time I heard this, I wanted to (somehow) drag my sorry state of a body to a mountaintop somewhere, scream as loud as I could for them to stop telling me that, and then fling myself over the side. Literally. I cringed every time I heard the phrase and would keep my distance from anyone who repeated it.

Few lines get me as heated as that one, especially when it comes from the faith community, because it's a complete crock of, well, you know . . .

If God *only* allowed in our life exactly what we could handle, we would have absolutely no reason or desire to reach out for help. We would think we were capable of doing *it all* based on our very own power, all the time, without divine help. We would be the master of our own universe and our own futures, effortlessly handling everything that came our way.

It doesn't work like that.

Everything I was experiencing was *way beyond* anything I could mentally or physically handle, and even if I mustered up every bit of power, it was a miserable fail. Every time. I could only get through this with God's strength, beyond what I could handle, beyond what I could muster. That, I believed, would guide me through the storm that raged around me.

As the events unraveled me, I began to realize that all of life would be a series of speed bumps and potholes and deep valleys for those of us who live with chronic illness. I knew that there would be places that I would be tested beyond my own strength (no matter what others assured me!), and I also knew that within that set of lessons was a growing understanding that I could put personal safeguards in place that could help as stressors hit and the signs of potential flares became clear. And the stressors *will* hit.

I discovered that my safeguards were numerous; for starters, rather than responding with a reactive and fearful mindset to life's events, I could retrain my brain and lean on my faith. When my stressors come and my cortisol levels are raised, that spikes an onset of symptoms within hours. Fevers, sores, rashes . . . you name it. Good to know.

Another key safeguard for me is being aware of my own tendency to let life's problems pull me into isolation and depression. Away from those who care for me, away from the God who seeks a relationship with me. And once I am separated from everyone who cares about me and left with my own spiraling thoughts, I get lost in a danger zone that becomes difficult to pull myself out of. My symptoms also increase as my body fights to find a balance against anxiety and worry. It took a long time for me to recognize the signs of this spiral starting—but now I have action plans in place that help prevent me from isolating myself.

Other safeguards relate to caring for my body. As I meet stressors, keeping my nutrition and diet at optimal levels (and eating regularly!) is, I've learned, nonnegotiable. While I am intentional and cognizant of each meal I am putting into my body, I tend to ramp up certain foods and herbs when I am met with intense stressors. I typically juice more: Lots of greens with ginger, lemon, and parsley. Lots of extra fresh fruits and vegetables, homemade soups, and bone broths. Items filled with probiotics, seeds, and healthy oils are added to additionally supplement my struggling body. Lysine to help counteract a mouth or nose full of lupus sores. Vitamin C to support the immune system. And herbs like licorice root, rehmannia, Chinese yam, and ashwagandha to support my adrenal glands and help my body have a healthier physiological response to stress. (Most of these were added through the help of a functional medicine physician I work with who specifically looked at the organ systems involved in my diagnoses and symptoms. I've been so helped by my work with a functional medicine doctor and a nutritionist that I recommend it for anyone needing a tailored supplement regimen specifically for their needs.)

I also learned it's important to create a small support team—my mom, Mickey, and key friends and family were willing to go the extra mile and help me during challenging times. For me, this was one of the most difficult safeguards to fully activate in my own life. It goes against my nature to ask people for help. I do not like feeling dependent on others. But the reality is, we aren't meant to do life alone, and we aren't designed to carry the heavy loads by ourselves. I was given friends and family for a reason. I have Jesus for a reason.

The last safeguard I discovered—and I'm still tweaking this to this very day—is continually learning ways to not only manage my stress but give my body the rest it needs regularly. It has taken years, but I have finally learned to say no, shut down the electronic devices, shut off the lights, and be present in peace and quiet. When I tell myself to just keep going and plow through (with caffeine in hand) is often when I need to put the caffeine down and let my body rest.

Everyone has different safeguards. Yours may be similar to mine or may be radically different, with therapies or solutions that work for your unique situation. And these safeguards will also likely change over time as your life changes and your disease state shifts. You'll become more in tune with your body and understand how stress affects you, and you'll discover what you need to remain balanced and as healthy as possible when a stressful event hits.

If you have never considered putting safeguards into place, you might begin now—before the next set of stressors hit. You might begin by first reflecting on how past stressful events have physically and mentally affected you (a journal can come in handy for recording your reflections). Maybe you went into a severe flare after you moved or started a new job. Perhaps you notice a trend of worsening fatigue and fevers when an unexpected stressful event occurs. Maybe you see a correlation between handling stress better and experiencing fewer symptoms. Or maybe you've discovered that when you've gotten the rest you've needed or faithfully taken helpful medications or followed a specific eating regimen that those stressors didn't quite turn your life upside down. Or maybe you learned that delegating tasks to people willing to help you free up time to rest correlated to a decrease in symptoms. You may have to dig a little here and fully detail or write out your needs when it comes to managing an illness on a daily basis. Having an emergency protocol for when one of life's surprises hits lessens the hit.

While severe flares can happen at times for people with autoimmune disease and chronic illness, you may notice you can lessen or shorten the duration of certain symptoms as you develop a plan to safeguard your health. In the years following my diagnosis, I didn't have any idea what protecting my health looked like. No one around me—not hospital staff, not rehab—ever mentioned safeguards. They didn't mention I might look for work-arounds or that I might start to pay attention to triggers and how my body tended to respond.

So it was in the year after Grandma died that I began to learn about these safeguards and how to balance severe symptoms with the challenges of career and household needs and a life with

Fabulous Finds

Journal Regularly

Journaling helps you recognize patterns and trends and helps you build safeguards and protocols to better manage your illness. Here are some things that make it into my daily journal:

- food and drink for each meal
- meds and supplements taken
- sun, heat, or cold exposure
- hours of sleep
- naps taken and length
- new foods or medicine I am trying
- daily symptoms I experience
- pain levels
- any travel or appointments
- stressors—good or bad
- menstrual cycle, if applicable
- exercise, if applicable
- alternative or complementary therapies used

my husband. Given the very basic task of taking care of myself, I felt completely incompetent. Much of that year was spent either in a hospital room or at home in my bedroom.

Even though this could have seemed like a limiting circumstance, as I faced new pressures in my career and new and different medical treatments, and as I was getting into a rhythm of a new marriage and still figuring out how to do life without my grandmother, I also craved time alone. In the solace of my bed, I found peace and quiet and a tranquil place where I could constantly talk to God. Life's violent storms felt like they were endlessly swirling, but I found a place of safety and silence in God and my pillow and the necessary rest.

When I look back on what I now call *my wilderness year*, I see it as a time of entering completely uncharted territory with no skills to navigate the challenges confronting me. Anyone with a new diagnosis will eventually feel this way. Every day was a balancing act, knowing that my survival depended on getting the balance right. With chronic illness, I never knew what was lurking around the corner, and I was still unaware of what measures were helping or hurting me.

All of us face wilderness seasons that can be scary and uncomfortable in all sorts of ways. But these seasons can also be liberating, and beautiful, and freeing. They offer us a place where we can find quiet and peace and time with God to listen to and have our character molded for future purposes that we are too limited to see just yet while in the wilderness.

We may not willingly enter into the wilderness (I went in basically kicking and screaming), but we know that it's a matter of time before we wind up there. And when we do, we know we're in good company. Jesus met one of his most difficult challenges when he entered the wilderness. Yet the Gospels record that he returned to these wild places. Why would he keep entering harsh, uncomfortable environments? When we read the Gospel texts, we see that it was in the wilderness that God prepared him for his future work. He entered the wild lands, time after time, and there—even with the challenges—found a period of peace, closeness with God, spiritual sustenance, and refinement.

The Bible relates that the process of refinement is directly related to trials. Several texts compare the process to refining gold, where in order to create a purer gold, it needs to be placed under intense heat, driving out the impurities mixed within.

And the refining process *is hot*.

And uncomfortable.

And oh so necessary.

When life applies heat to us in a variety of ways, our weaknesses, and faults, and struggles—our impurities—are exposed. But as the fire grows in intensity, we are able to be part of the divine burning off of those things that hinder our lives. And through the fire, on the other side, we emerge stronger, more refined.

At first in that year, I didn't correlate how my illness and medical issues would be crucial to my growth and the way my life was being refined. When we are constantly in pain, fatigued, emotionally and physically drained, and feeling like we are losing control of our health, we can respond in all sorts of ways. Illness can sometimes make us cranky, sad, snappy, irritable, unmotivated—and just ready to give up. And truthfully, chronic illness wasn't bringing out my best side. I felt like a new version of the seven dwarfs fable: crabby, achy, sleepy, snippy, rashy, sweaty, and just straight bitchy all rolled into one.

But for me, chronic illness became the heat God used to show me I had major control issues: I thought could handle everything on my own. It took a long time for me to accept that I actually only have a very small amount of control over my body and my life in general. For years I had tried to control every little thing. And for years it kept tripping me up. It felt like carrying sand in my hands 24/7 while trying not to let even a grain slip between the cracks of my fingers—a losing battle.

The year after Grandma passed was gloomy, and heart-breaking, and lonely. Everything in my life shifted suddenly. I went from growing up living with my grandmother and having daily interactions with her to now moving away to a new setting while married, facing a foreign set of health challenges, and no longer having her to turn to in a shared kitchen space or after hours there, sitting next to each other and talking as she had her espresso and pastries. My new home was quiet and somewhat lonely each day, as my husband was away at work for long hours. I craved the safety and stability she represented. I craved the comfort she brought to me each day and our friendship.

But God was calling me to find a different kind of safety and peace and stability and comfort. And with Grandma no longer there, I looked for an endless source of that stability and found it in God. When I found out about the blood clot that went to my lung, and the brain aneurysm, and as I continued to return to the hospital and then finally hired a nurse to come to my home each week to help bathe me and assist me in exercising, and as I sat for hours crying and staring at that first chemo pill I was terrified to swallow, I ran to God, with my fear, and doubt and frustration, and sometimes a really crappy attitude. And I kept saying, whispering, screaming out, "Here's my life, God. You can have it all!"

Because it was too heavy for me.

It was too heavy for my husband.

And it was too heavy for my mom.

And none of us were designed to carry these burdens all alone.

As each unexpected health event, or life hiccup, or challenge in my marriage or career occurred, I shared it with God and sat back in wonderment at God's using every circumstance as the fire got hotter to mold me into a less doubtful, more faithful, less resentful, more grateful, less crabby, more joyful person.

Slowly I began to notice a decrease in anxiety about the "what ifs" and more growing excitement about the moments of breakthrough I was seeing in my career and marriage and health. Instead of the wilderness seeming so scary, in time it became an adventure; even when I didn't know the path, I felt I was being led by the One who was with me.

By allowing God to step out ahead of me on the unknown path, I was guided through dangerous territory. When the load I carried was too heavy, I learned to rest in knowing God carried me and the load.

Whenever I spend time in the wilderness now, I hold onto those things I've learned:

> Remember that none of the challenges you have faced or will face are wasted by the Divine hand. The lessons learned through this time, the resiliency you build—it will all be used when you meet a future challenge or will be shared with others who are just starting out on their wilderness journey and are in need of support and encouragement.
>
> Whenever you spend time in the wilderness, you are being shaped and refined in ways unique to that moment. And as trying as wilderness seasons can be, it is only through these life experiences where you undergo metamorphoses that you emerge stronger, more patient, wiser, and kinder.

When you emerge, you will gain trust that God has helped you through that moment and that even more in future moments, you will be cared for, carried. You will begin to lean on the understanding that with the Divine beside you, you will never journey through the wild on your own.

These nuggets I have learned in the past help me meet challenging seasons and hold out hope for the future.

And as new opportunities are put in my path, and as I meet others currently in their wilderness or in the painful, purifying fire, I know I can share my story about clinging to faith instead of fear in the middle of life's unknowns. I can tell them how I was refined, shaped, and loved on while on this wilderness path and how it prepared me for the future life seasons I was about to walk into. And I truly believe a similar story is going to play out in your life, even though it may be too far in the distance at the moment for you to see it clearly now.

You *will* emerge from the fire, the wild path, the badlands, and the wastelands—these sacred lands—a warrior. And you will share your scars and bruises and triumphs and wins with the next person about to journey into the unknown. And you will know yourself on an intimate level, recognizing your strength with a newfound confidence that you can and will survive any wilderness life throws at you in the future.

Bourbon Cold-Busting Tea

Prep/Cook Time: 5–7 minutes
Method: Teakettle
Yield: 1 serving

Bourbon has long been a go-to home remedy when dealing with the inevitable cold, as it is said to help relieve nasal congestion. This bourbon cold-busting tea is my "adult" beverage when I am struggling with a cold and have a scratchy sore throat and stuffy nose and just feel all-around miserable. The

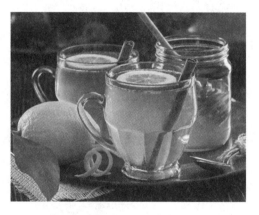

peppermint tea bag and whole cinnamon stick gives this tea just the kick it needs, and the warmth and honey soothe a sore throat. For the bourbon, I use Woodford Reserve, but you can use any brand you like.

INGREDIENTS

1 bag peppermint tea
1–2 ounces bourbon (2 to 4 tablespoons)
1 cinnamon stick
1 heaping teaspoon honey
Juice from half of 1 lemon

Bring 8–10 ounces of water to a boil in a teakettle. Combine peppermint tea bag, bourbon, a cinnamon stick, honey, and lemon juice in a mug. Pour boiling water into mug and let steep for 3–4 minutes. Sip, relax, and get ready for a great rest.

TWELVE

My Kitchen, My Situation Room

*The food you eat can be either the safest
and most powerful form of medicine
or the slowest form of poison.*
                                                    —Ann Wigmore

It took over a year from the time my grandmother passed away for me to feel like the wilderness season I had entered was finally coming to a close. My major health emergencies quieted down and were better controlled, my journalism career was holding at a steady pace (which had me over the moon), and Mickey and I developed a comfortable rhythm with one another in our marriage.

And then something unexpected happened.

For the first time since Grandma's death, I suddenly had this overwhelming desire to get back in the kitchen and get my hands dirty. At first, the feeling was foreign to me. It had been so long. But as I returned to my beloved kitchen, I realized that something was marinating deep within, now ready to come out. In that enthusiasm came an epiphany: no longer did I see food in the same way.

Being in the wilderness season for so long, my ideas around chronic illness, nourishment, and what feeds us shifted to an entirely different level. On the spiritual level, I understood that without a daily connection to God, I couldn't maintain my strength, so I relied on an ongoing relationship with Divine help. I also began to reflect that if we're not continually consuming nourishing foods, our body becomes weaker—and that we need daily nourishment to fight chronic illness.

A stronger version of myself emerged, with increased mental clarity and more overall energy. Inspired by a return to the kitchen, I once again began to immerse myself in researching the correlations between diet, nutrition, and chronic illness / autoimmune diseases. To my surprise, information in these areas had grown exponentially from just a few years prior when I first began this endeavor. To better grasp the landscape of nutrition and create a plan of attack for my body and the symptoms that plagued me, I reenlisted the help of the nutritionist, allergist, and functional medicine physician I had worked with before.

I wanted to know what strategies and tactics I needed to incorporate to help me win this battle going on in my body. And I felt this team of trusted advisors and experts were part of the strategy to find the answers. In my mind, we all played valuable roles in what I called "Operation Healing." I was excited to see what the future held. As my medication regimen got sorted out and things calmed down in my body, I shifted my focus to the elements of right foods. And even if a full and complete healing wasn't in the cards, I was on a mission to take back the "territory" that had been taken from me.

One particular day, I walked down my staircase and headed toward the kitchen. Stopping just before I entered, I scanned the space in its entirety as I had done from the staircase some time ago. But this time, it felt different.

Hope was present here.

Now, instead of being reminded of death and loss, I saw new potential and life-giving opportunities. I saw the possibility of restoration in my body. The kitchen became a laboratory of sorts, where I began to carry out numerous experiments and discover some of my greatest work toward healing my body.

My first plan of attack was to "Can the Crap"—an event where every cupboard, cabinet, refrigerator shelf, and drawer was cleaned out and unloaded of any type of food or drink that wasn't fueling or nourishing to my body. For me, this basically meant saying goodbye to processed and boxed foods, sugar-filled foods like cookies and chocolate (my favorites), and anything loaded with chemicals or a long list of ingredients I couldn't even pronounce. I trained my eye. If the ingredient list was lines long and took up a good portion of the container or box, in the garbage it went. I wanted fresh, pure, nutrient-dense, life-giving foods to provide my body with the fuel it so desperately longed for.

If someone had handed me a cup of brominated vegetable oil and said to drink it, I would have looked at them as though they had ten heads. And if they had handed me a spoonful of red #4 and said, "Down the hatch, Marisa," I would have flat out refused. So why had I been willing to overlook ingredients like these in the past and allow them entry into my kitchen, let alone into my precious, delicate body? *No more*, I promised myself.

After the "Can the Crap" phase was complete, I sat down with my allergist and went over results from both the extensive bloodwork and the skin tests I recently completed at her office. If you aren't aware, there is a high correlation between people with allergies and allergic diseases and increased rates of autoimmune disease (the research is actually fascinating).[1]

With more knowledge under my belt about how my body—and my overactive immune system—was now reacting to certain foods, I began the process of reworking some of my favorite family recipes into adapted recipes containing ingredients that were safe and healthier for my body.

My grocery lists also underwent a major upheaval.

Growing up in an Italian household means there's an endless supply of wheat and dairy in almost every meal. Turns out, my body is not fond of either—in addition to a long list of other food items that often show up in the Italian kitchen. I won't bore you with the list. But as newfound knowledge began with the development of new recipes and work-arounds, I soon was enjoying the meals I grew up on and loved. The ones that brought back a lifetime of memories with just one whiff of their aroma.

This season of kitchen experimentation was truly a blessing in my life, as it coincided with a phase in my health and food journalism career that was picking up speed. I was able to take the research I was already doing for myself related to how different foods react in people living with autoimmune disease and chronic illness and create recipes or disseminate findings to others in the same situation, bringing them some level of healing for their bodies.

The next two years flowed with experimentation, the development of new recipes, and adjustments in food regimens as I learned what worked for my body. Whole foods were in, and processed foods were out; homemade bone broth became a staple; I dove heavily into juicing—to the point where I began teaching a class in my town. I worked with my functional medicine doctor to align the different regimens: prescription medications, nutritional supplements, and diet. Collagen? Yes. Turmeric, black pepper, and fresh ginger? You guessed it. And probiotics? Double-check. In fact, I looked at different probiotic strains to see which ones my gut actually lacked rather than throwing a random probiotic supplement at my gut issues. This required comprehensive stool tests at independent laboratories. As I began to make headway in developing the right cocktail of all the above, I met with increasing progress.

My hair stopped falling out as much—no more clumps on the pillow and in my hands during a shower. There weren't as many urticaria (hives) outbreaks happening on my body. I gained needed weight and strength. While I still needed naps, there weren't as many, and for the most part, I was sleeping better. One of the biggest changes in the new mix of regimens was the increase in my energy levels. No longer was I hitting the wall an hour or so after waking up in the morning. Where once just having breakfast and getting dressed would send crushing fatigue throughout my body, now I had more sustained strength. And hours of it.

Each of these little successes accumulated, and for the first time in a long while, I could feel this vibration of life flowing through my veins again. At random moments, I would look up and just start in with excitement and gratitude to God, acknowledging my earlier doubts that I would ever progress to this point. I'd come a long way since that traumatic day where I lay in a hospital bed, completely broken, being informed by a rheumatologist that I had an incurable disease.

Again, hope was now present here.

Now, after living with lupus and several other autoimmune diseases for almost two decades, I've witnessed a radical shift in how society has grown to value nutrition and taken an increasingly open-minded attitude toward understanding the foods we digest and how crucial the right foods are in supporting and fueling the chronically ill body.

I've also grown in my own understanding of how many people living with chronic illness and autoimmune disease typically have multiple issues, often referred to as overlap diseases. No longer do I subscribe to the belief that there is one all-encompassing diet that will work for everyone. In fact, I'm no longer a fan of the word *diet* either. It conjures up images of deprivation from foods we love, and it adds to stress as well as a fear of failure when we don't stick to it. Plus, it has the word *die* in it, which rubs me the wrong way. I've cheated death too many times to count.

Now I only want to surround myself with things that speak life into my body and my mind. Instead of a diet, I've begun recommending individuals create a *food protocol,* starting with a life-fueling food plan, for a source of constant energy and nutrients. And just as no two bodies are the same, no two protocols will be the same.

Among my friends are those who have health and autoimmune issues. One friend who has lupus and Hashimoto's disease has decreased the severity of her symptoms and increased her energy by creating a food protocol unique to her set of conditions. Another friend who has lupus, diabetes, and celiac disease has gotten positive results with a completely different protocol. No matter what your health challenges are, I have no doubt that you'll eventually find a life-fueling food, rest, and exercise regimen that will be specific to your needs—with time and a heck of a lot of effort and through detailed journaling, allergy tests, independent lab gut/stool tests, and work with nutritionists, food coaches, and/or an allergist. It's trial and error, but it is completely worth it.

This is your life we are talking about. Fight for it.

The greatest piece of advice I can offer you as you step forth into your food journey is to be unbelievably patient with yourself *and* the process. It's been years, and I am still learning new ways to support and heal my body every single day. It also requires ongoing readjustment. Some supplements and food regimens that helped me in the past don't provide me with those same dramatic results today. I've also learned that the various seasons of my life—particularly those in which I'm in a flare—require different food and supplementation regimens, as I previously mentioned. You'll most likely have a daily protocol and a ramped-up flare protocol too.

Taking this road requires being completely committed to the process of trial and error. Out of five new supplements, foods, or protocols you try, only one may actually work for you and provide a physical or mental benefit. Instead of viewing this as four failures, look at it as having one more thing to add to your specific healing protocol.

Make sure to take copious notes on everything that works for you in a journal you've set apart for your healing journey. Detail how you've applied ideas, how you've made use of supplements, what effect they've had, what symptoms may have decreased, and everything related to your body's response.

For those tempted to try all five supplements or food protocols at once, it's best to stick with one thing at a time. Try it out fully and notice how your body reacts to it. Trying everything all at once makes it difficult to find out what isn't working and why when your body has a poor reaction.

I've said it several times already, but it can't be stressed enough: journaling is your friend in this process. Actually, your bestie. Grab a cheap notebook from the dollar store and keep a daily log of everything you eat, drink, and ingest, whether it is a new medication, supplement, herb, and so on. Notate how you feel throughout the day and rate your energy levels continuously.

Keep checking in with yourself on your body's response. Did you feel more energetic after you took that licorice root supplement or exhausted after you ate something loaded with white flour? Do you continually notice a small patch of hives or a rash after you ingest eggs, corn, or soy? Is there an increase in symptoms around your menstrual cycle? Did you notice a fever or rash after you were in the direct sun? These are the types of answers you are searching for. No matter what you are eating, doing, or trying—document *all of it*.

In addition to practicing patience with yourself, committing to shifting your mindset about food and your kitchen is imperative—and it may not be as easy as you think. Consider what runs through your mind when you step into your kitchen. How do you feel mentally and physically when you are in a flare-up, feverish, and crabby and you know you have to eat or make yourself a meal?

When we are drowning in a sea of fatigue and frustration and pain, it can be really difficult to not see food prep or cooking as a chore or just as something we want to get over with as soon as possible, not caring if we go to bed that night hungry or we have to eat a piece of old bread or our kid's leftover Pop-Tart.

I challenge you to shift your thinking and begin seeing illness as a battlefield and your kitchen as your situation room—a place where you can plan ways to have a good offense for the war taking place inside your body. When you can get to the situation room early (before a flare, say), you can develop your plan of action for the times you don't have energy.

But there will be times you straight-up feel like you are in the midst of a flare. That's when utilizing your kitchen in the right ways offers you an opportunity to give your body the nutrients and energy it desperately needs. After we are diagnosed with an autoimmune disease or chronic illness, there comes a point of realization that our relationship with food has to change. And another point when we realize our relationship with food *has* changed. And while we can still absolutely eat for pleasure and enjoyment, we understand, admit, and commit to the fact that we are eating for survival and healing.

When I talk about healing, it's important to understand that it's deep work—not slightly changing your diet and adding in a few supplements and you're magically healed overnight. That is a myth. It requires attention, journaling, and the development of food, supplement, and medical protocols. And it requires frequent returns to the situation room. That's not to say we can't experience supernatural healing. Or that we can't experience a certain level of healing when it comes to our food intake. The results will differ for everyone. And even if you don't see major wins right away, I just want to encourage you to continue moving forward in this process. Remember, countless small wins add up and can change your life over time.

I found—in addition to the physical benefits I briefly described earlier—that within a few years of really experimenting with various food protocols and making my own regimen, I was able to decrease my number of prescription medications—from twelve down to a range of two to four at any given time. I wasn't able to get off of *all* of my medications, but being able to drop more than a half dozen was a huge win in my book!

So how will you initiate this plan of attack when it comes to food and nutrition and healing your body? This answer looks different for everyone. Personally, I went through years of trial and error, and I committed several months of my life to every food protocol I was willing to try, taking abundant notes as the experiment ensued. With limited finances, I rationed the money I had available for allergist visits to discover my allergies and sensitivities and also for a small number of visits to a nutritionist and my functional medicine doctor to get the big picture of my health issues and possible solutions. As a plan began to form, I then reallocated those tight funds to solely go toward supplements, food shopping, herbs, and other functional medicine products (with the occasional follow-up appointment).

I spent a tremendous amount of time researching and studying different food protocols and then planning a dedicated amount of time to trying each one. And the personal experiments were numerous, consisting of raw foods and juicing, to paleo, to the autoimmune protocol, to the anti-inflammatory diet, to the leaky gut protocol, to veganism, to intermittent

Fabulous Finds

Developing a Strategy

What does your situation room's strategy look like? You may want to consider specific food plan options such as anti-inflammatory, paleo, or leaky gut if your focus is on improving specific symptoms. Or you can create your own food plan by considering what your most debilitating symptoms are each day, making a protocol with food and supplementation, and working with a nutritionist or functional medicine doctor to try to decrease these symptoms. Chart it out—take it one step at a time—and make a commitment each day to record detailed notes. Symptoms are the enemy here so take time detailing your plan of attack before you step into battle.

fasting, and more. With each regimen, I documented the different positive benefits I reaped, creating a unique system of healing for my body.

My refrigerator became filled with countless containers of berries, fresh fruits, cruciferous vegetables, fermented foods, and fresh herbs like parsley, sage, and rosemary. I feel like everywhere you looked in my kitchen, you would come across fresh ginger root and turmeric; freshly cut, massive aloe leaves; coconut oil; and jars of raw honey. There was always a slow cooker brewing up some flavor of homemade bone broth, a juicer on the counter, and bags of quinoa, millet, and black rice. I feel like I drank my weight in green tea, green juices, and nutrient-dense soups and stews. During the day, I snacked on roasted vegetables, seeds, and fresh dates. And no matter what I ate or drank or which supplement I ingested, it all went into its allotted place in my journal. In some sense, it was almost a full-time job, but the payment I received from it was the best payment of all, worth far more than any numerical amount: it was giving me my life back.

Through analyzing the years of data and notes from my journals, I saw clear patterns of what helped my body flourish and what sent my body backward—and whether it affected my physical or mental health. Though I didn't see its value at the beginning, as I returned to these journals time and time again, I began to realize how crucial they were in helping me save myself.

Your relationship with food is *the longest relationship* you are going to have in your entire life. From the minute you were born, your survival relied upon it. And now, living with a chronic illness, your life depends on it in a very different way. So step into your kitchen and own it! Say to your kitchen, "What happens in here is going to radically show up as a beneficial shift within my body!" And as you take the foods from your kitchen, with every morsel that goes into your mouth, remember that promise and ask yourself, "Is this giving me life or sending me backward?" And, yes, when you have a bad day and need to throw caution to the wind, when you just want something cozy and sweet and delicious, have some options on hand of your favorite things—but the work-around version, the healthy version. Don't throw away all of your hard work and energy during a momentary challenge.

Experiment with foods and drinks and supplements you've never tried before. Explore healing spices like ginger, cinnamon, turmeric, and cloves by adding them to drinks and dishes and warm teas. Research a variety of different food protocols that you might be willing to try—like the anti-inflammatory diet, autoimmune protocol, paleo, keto, leaky gut, grain-free, and so on—and set a dedicated time frame to the research in order to discover if you notice a beneficial effect.

For each new endeavor, each new stage of research, I would give each day to God, and every morning I would ask for increased wisdom to discern what could help my body, what would provide mental and physical energy to help throughout this endeavor. My prayer was for the Divine's help to discover the information I needed to make the best decision about my health—including what I was eating/drinking and supplements I was about to try—and to guide the doctors I was working with. I prayed—and continue to pray—that God would lead me to the people who could help me on this journey.

As you build a stronger foundation in the area of food and understand how it affects your physical and mental health, don't forget to continue to feed your spiritual health. Be present in the moments you are cooking and eating. Take time each day to sit in stillness, mentally scan your body, and ask yourself how you are feeling. Consider your headspace. You can feed your body

Fabulous Finds

Speak Life

Remember to #SpeakLife in, through, and over yourself during the battle. Here's my #SpeakLife list:

- I will provide my body with as much nourishment as possible as it fights this battle.
- I will celebrate small wins.
- I will not allow frustration to swallow me whole if this process takes longer than I expected.
- I will listen to and allow the Divine to lead me to various sources of healing that I may be currently unaware of.
- I will step out of my comfort zone to find new ways to nourish my body.
- I will alter my plan of action or try multiple approaches to find the healing I am seeking.
- I will remember that no matter the outcome, I am loved, worthy, safe—and I am a warrior.

the most life-nourishing foods possible, but if you feel alone or angry, if you have no hope or believe you have no purpose, these depleting thoughts will have an overall effect on how you feel physically. Meditate, pray, and find your own spiritual road that provides comfort, support, and love. As you do, you will strengthen both the physical and the spiritual body—nourished by faith, nourished by food. For when we lean into the truth of a healing hope, we discover new ways to live.

RECIPE

Easy Energy Bites

Prep Time: 5 minutes
Method: Food processor
Yield: 10–12 balls, about 1 inch in diameter

Being a warrior and learning to #SpeakLife over yourself are important. They take energy. Fatigue is one of my biggest challenges when it comes to living with a chronic illness, so these energy bites come in handy on the tough days when I have a long list of must-do doctor appointments and so on. They are very quick and easy to make, delicious, and quite filling. I always have some on hand in my refrigerator, as they make a healthy and yummy snack.

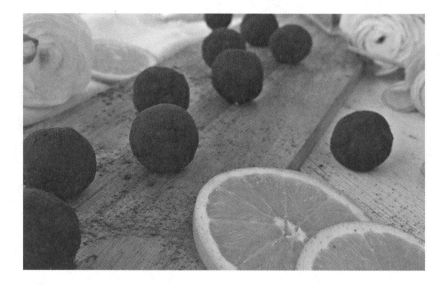

INGREDIENTS

⅓ cup shelled sunflower seeds
9–10 fresh dates, pitted and cut in half
¼ cup raisins
Dash or two or cinnamon
Shredded or desiccated coconut
1 tablespoon warm water
1 tablespoon collagen powder, optional

Place sunflower seeds in food processor and pulse a few times to partially grind them up (but don't grind them into a flour). Add dates, raisins, cinnamon, and collagen powder if using. Pulse for a few seconds and then use the blend button until everything is well combined. Remove food processor lid and test stickiness of the mixture. Mixture should be sticky enough to roll into balls. If mixture is too dry, add a tablespoon of warm water, cover food processor, and blend again to mix well.

Roll individual balls about an inch or so wide. Finish by rolling each ball in coconut and enjoy!

THIRTEEN

Speak All of Your Truth

A small body of determined spirits fired
by an unquenchable faith in their mission
can alter the course of history.
                              —Mahatma Gandhi

Chronic illness, trauma, and trials can teach us an awful lot about ourselves—good and bad. But in this chapter, we're going to focus on the good. The following are among the lessons we can learn from these experiences:

- We learn to be kinder to our body.
- We learn to be compassionate to others who have their own set of struggles.
- We learn patience and begin to understand that healing is not linear and can take time.
- We learn how to advocate for ourselves and our body.

- We get an intimate lesson in judgment and how what we see on the outside tells almost none of the story of what someone has endured.
- We typically recognize at some point just how resilient we really are.

If you are anything like me, you want to contemplate those lessons and take all those experiences you've survived and discern what to do with them. When it comes to "trials and tribulations," I tend to look for the bigger purpose. Surely there is a reason for this—or multiple good things that can come from this. Perhaps that reason is to help someone else—or at least that's usually my first thought nowadays.

After emerging from the fire, my prayer is usually one of gratitude, followed by "God, is there some way you want me to use the lessons I've learned? How?"

I listen for something that tugs on my heart that tells me these experiences have a larger purpose. Sometimes as I wait for an answer, it usually comes as I look at all the ways God equips me—and each of us—in a unique way to share what's been learned and to use resources gained in a difficult time to help the lives of others. For me, that unique path of helping others has come through food journalism, social media posts, and sharing resources with communities that advocate for people struggling with immune issues.

For some of you, your platform may be sharing your story online through a blog or web article, while for others, your gift is the spoken word or another form of creative work. Maybe you venture into the area of creating vlogs or a YouTube channel, teaching your own course, or speaking on stage to hundreds or thousands of people. Maybe you will become a whirlwind force in the chronically ill community. Or perhaps you will write a book

Fabulous Finds

The Battle Cry List

Write down at least five positive things you have learned since your trial or diagnosis—these could be general things or things you've specifically learned about yourself. Keep this list and return to it when you are having a challenging moment, or add to it. This will become your battle cry when life wants to throw opposition your way.

or share your story in some other form. In some distinct way, you have been challenged, and you have also been gifted. What that gift is, is yours to share. It doesn't have to be big or extravagant; it may be helping a friend struggling with a new diagnosis over a cup of tea where you can privately share what you've learned and offer life-encouraging words.

We weren't put on the earth for only ourselves, for only our health; we were meant to be in community and help all of creation find healing. We live in a time where society—and especially those on social media—is quick to judge or condemn rather than help someone who is struggling. But when we offer hope, encouragement, and a helping hand, it changes things. There are a lot of hurting people who can use life-giving words spoken into their world. Think back to when someone offered you a word of hope when you were just starting out on your chronic illness journey. Pay it forward and help deliver hope to someone in the trenches, someone utterly exhausted, someone about to give up. We just need to open ourselves up and let our experiences not only help us but help others.

When I first started LupusChick.com, I was thrilled if four or five people a week visited and read my blog. (Of course, most of those people in the beginning were my family members and close friends!) They supported me in my small endeavor, and that support, in addition to believing God was leading me to do this, gave me fuel to keep going. I wanted to reach more people, though, and being new to both blogging and the writing world at the time, I had zero idea about how to do that.

It just so happened—and I call it a God-incidence—that around the same time I was building up the blog, my husband and I had read a prayer—the Prayer of Jabez—from the Bible. We began to pray it multiple times a day:

> Oh, that You would bless me indeed, and enlarge my territory, that Your hand would be with me, and that You would keep me from evil, that I may not cause pain. (adapted)

As I prayed that prayer, I wanted to focus on the blessings that came from God and not just my endeavors. I prayed for an expanded territory—for me that means a way in which the blessings I was given and the story I had to tell could grow and be shared in ways that would bless others and offer them hope. I prayed for blessings and restoration, if God meant those things for me. And I prayed that I would never be a source of pain for the people God put in my life.

Now, I don't know if it was specifically this prayer or that I was spending more time praying that my experience would be a help to others, but soon I was bewildered and amazed at the incredible things that started happening in my life—and especially with LupusChick—in just those first few years. Our monthly social reach went from about fifteen thousand people per month to almost five hundred thousand people per month, and our social media accounts started growing like wildfire. My small blog got a makeover and became a full-fledged website for everything lupus and autoimmune disease.

Completely unexpected in this time, I was titled Mrs. Rochester in the Mrs. America pageant system. And I also started working with government officials in my county of New York, where May was officially named Lupus Awareness Month. LupusChick kept growing, and we filed for and received nonprofit status. My heart in all of this was not just to educate people on lupus and autoimmune disease but to somehow tangibly help those who were struggling so much and needed a way to financially support themselves and afford medications specific to their condition—medications that were often costly.

God brought incredible donors my way—people I had never met, and I had no idea how they heard about us. With the first monies that were donated, we were able to gift ten people with partial funding to return to a trade or certification program that would ultimately help them financially support themselves.

Other doors began to open. I had told God something on my heart was speaking, though I had no idea how to begin. But soon I was invited to speak. At first, it was in nearby cities to small rooms of twenty or thirty people, telling portions of my life story and talking about aspects of living with chronic illness. This grew into traveling across the United States, delivering keynote speeches at medical schools and galas, raising money to help others, and sharing that no matter how hopeless or lost their current life season seemed, there was hope. New opportunities followed in magazines and on television, each one a vehicle to share, educate, and make even just one more person feel like they weren't in this battle alone. The LupusChick story was even featured as the thirty-fifth chapter in Lady Gaga's new book, *Channel Kindness*.

But perhaps my greatest eye-opening experience of how God was using my experiences to help another person came a few years ago. I spoke at a Mrs. New York event (I was titled Mrs. New York Universal in 2015) as part of the US Universal pageant system. As I was walking down a quiet hallway, returning from the restroom, all of a sudden I heard, "LupusChick! Oh my goodness, you're LupusChick!" Someone who didn't know my name recognized me as LupusChick, the name I felt God had given me in a dream. In the three minutes we talked, she spilled out her own story, saying, "One night after nights of contemplating how I was going to take my life, I found your website. And I started reading the blogs and your story. And I clicked to the Facebook page and read hundreds of comments from all these other women who were going through exactly what I was going through, and for the first time in so long, I thought, *OMG, I am not alone.* This isn't a death sentence. There may just be hope here. And it was the first time my mind shifted away from ending my life."

My measly little—hideous-looking, if we're being real—blog that had only a few readers in its first few months eventually played a part in helping someone step back from the brink of killing themselves—and into hope?

That conversation—one of many through the years—continues to fuel my fire in the moments I am completely exhausted and feel like I may not have the power to go forward. With God's strength and the realization that one person putting themselves out there and doing something tangible to help others can actually change lives provides me with a supernatural strength that even lupus can't tear down.

After I walked away from that conversation, God reminded me that everything we say, everything we utter to ourselves, to the world, to the people who hear our story can speak life or can speak death into the mind and heart. And in that moment for this young woman, the stories I shared and the hundreds of truth-filled comments she read from hundreds of strangers on a website were enough to speak such life into her and the despair she felt that her thoughts shifted to hope.

What is it you put out into the world, into your neighborhood—what experiences and insights can you bring that can serve the greater good? Your words have the ability to alter someone's life forever. It can seem a little intimidating at first, but stay with it. Stay rooted in faith, knowing that you were put here for such a time as this. When your moment comes to step out and spread love and life, don't be afraid to use your voice and speak your story, your truth. Don't be afraid to be heard. The world can't get *your* story, and your insight, and your hope from *anyone* else.

The world needs to hear your story, that story that grew like that seed in the dark soil, when everything felt like it was buried. Even if you feel you don't know how to speak your story, the One who is the ground of all being will help you find your voice, refining you from within and ultimately helping you use your voice to help someone else find theirs.

And when you use your voice for good, you build your words on a foundation of authenticity and honesty, relating your life story and experiences. This is when you can see the real life-changing magic happen. When I first started LupusChick, I stayed really surface-y. I was afraid of offending anyone, grossing someone out with too many medical details, or getting too personal, and I didn't want to sound like I was whining or complaining. I edited my voice so much that it sounded nothing like me. And I saw I wasn't connecting with people. So one day in prayer I felt like God was encouraging me to get authentic and put it out there, the way I did in my everyday life with friends and family—no filter and brutally honest.

So I shared it all—the good, the bad, the ugly, and the absolutely mortifying. I shared the things I thought I would never, ever share. And instantly, people became more engaged. I learned that speaking all of your truth—even the really hard, messy, and awkward parts, the ones you want to forget about completely—and sharing the growth you've endured and the ways you've lived into hope allows others to envision what could be possible for them, what a future season may hold, after their current trial by fire passes.

No matter how our raw, detailed, sometimes dark story may end (because let's face it, trials don't always end with rainbows and unicorns), we can share that despite it all, we walked through that trial with hope, with God, with our community. Speak what you know and what you have experienced in full honesty and in faith, and watch as lives around you change, hold onto hope, and find strength to pass on the spark.

Remember the story of Job, how he prayed and praised God even when he felt like he was losing every life-giving thing?

Share your grief, and persecutions, and hardships, and winning moments, and suffering. Speak up for others who aren't being heard, who don't have the energy to advocate for themselves. Speak up for those experiencing utter despair in this moment, those too sick to speak up and fight for themselves.

Use the life you are blessed with to *speak* life to others—in every way possible.

Turkey (or Chicken) Cornbread

Prep Time: 15 minutes

Cook Time: 40 minutes total

Method: Stovetop and oven

Yield: 6 servings

Among the things my life is blessed with is food, and one of the ways that I #SpeakLife to family and friends and those in the LupusChick community is through my shared recipes. Here's one that I know for sure will not leave one crumb on the dinner table! Whenever I have leftover turkey and gravy from the holidays or enough rotisserie chicken on hand, I always make this cornbread. When it comes to the corn muffin mix, I use Jiffy Vegetarian (because it has minimal ingredients) with a flax egg. Just remember to cut yourself a slice first when you pull it out of the oven, because it won't last long.

INGREDIENTS

Filling

3 tablespoons butter (or butter alternative)

1 yellow onion, diced

¾ cup carrots, diced

¾ cup fennel bulb, diced (substitute celery if you do not have fennel)

¼ teaspoon salt

¼ teaspoon pepper

½ teaspoon dried thyme

½ teaspoon nutmeg

½ teaspoon ground sage

4 cups leftover turkey or rotisserie chicken (fully cooked and ripped apart or shredded)

1¼ cups gravy (if you don't have leftover gravy from a holiday meal, try Imagine's roasted turkey gravy)

Topping
1 box corn muffin mix, prepared as per instructions
1 can corn, rinsed and drained
8 ounces shredded cheddar cheese or cheese substitute

One 5 × 9 baking dish

Preheat oven to 400°F. Grease a 5 × 9 baking dish well. In a large saucepan, melt butter or butter alternative over medium heat. Add diced onion, carrots, fennel, salt, pepper, thyme, nutmeg, and sage. Cook vegetables and spices uncovered until the vegetables are soft, about 8 to 10 minutes. Turn off the heat and stir in the leftover turkey or chicken. Pour the meat-and-vegetable mixture into the greased baking dish and even out with spoon. Pour the gravy evenly over the meat and vegetables. Set aside and begin to prepare the topping.

In a separate bowl, prepare your corn muffin mix according to the package—use a flax egg if you don't want to add an actual egg. Add drained corn and cheese to the prepared muffin mixture and mix well. Pour over the meat and vegetables in the baking dish and spread evenly with a spoon. Bake on middle rack, uncovered for 25 to 30 minutes or until golden brown and a fork or toothpick comes out clean.

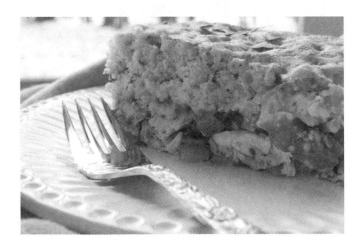

FOURTEEN

What It Means to Be Made Whole

Breathe, darling. This is just a chapter.
It's not your whole story.

—S. C. Lourie

Most of us think about healing as related to an illness or about our bodies, but one of the greatest things I've witnessed over the year is a healing of both my heart and my thinking—and my relationship to food and my kitchen. When I was created, God knew I'd have a special affinity for food—creating it, touching it, combining it in unique ways, and experiencing enjoyment when people would partake in the foods I made. You might even say that interacting with food is one of my love languages. It's like gift giving. You see, I love giving presents so much that I can't even wait until the specific occasion to give someone my gift for them. But what I love even more than giving gifts is cooking or baking for people and then sitting back and watching them indulge and enjoy themselves.

Over these years, God has helped my heart heal. As it healed, I rediscovered my love for the kitchen after Grandma passed away. I was reminded that despite the expanse of the earth and the universe and losses and separations, incredible magic can occur right within the four walls of that special room in my home. In the kitchen, stories will continue to be shared, memories created, heartbreaks healed, relationships strengthened, secrets told, recipes created, and physical bodies rejuvenated. Not only was my broken heart healed, but in years of trial and error around developing the best recipes for my body, I gained a kitchen wisdom that led to my having even more energy to physically spend time in the place that has brought—and continues to bring—me immense pleasure.

Now on the good days, you can find me spending my free time in the kitchen, countertops loaded with ingredients and spices. Appliances whirring, worship music or '80s tunes blaring on high (don't judge; I may or may not be addicted to old George Michael and Prince tunes), pen and paper for notes, my camera nearby, and my rescue dog waiting by the kitchen entrance hoping a morsel drops on the floor (and by drop, I mean the dog knows his human is a sucker for his adorable face and accidentally-on-purpose will let a piece of food "fall" in his direction).

Perhaps I'm drawn back to the kitchen again and again because it is there I feel God is present as well as my grandmother. Every single time I show up, I know they are company.

It is in the kitchen that I find peace and calm and hope.

And it is here I feel a magical electricity in the air—a currency of potential for further learning and experimentation and growth—that I know brings healing to my body somehow.

As I continue to live with chronic illness, the perspective I bring to each day as I enter the kitchen is an acknowledgment that the things that have brought me healing here—Jesus and food and the love of my grandmother and the shared meals with family—have helped me survive and thrive.

What I've learned in the kitchen about how food nourishes a body challenged by illness, I've also discovered in scripture, from its earliest verses. That the Divine created food as a gift to give us both enjoyment and sustenance, as he said to Noah: "Every moving thing that lives shall be food for you; and just as I gave you the green plants, I give you everything" (Genesis 9:3).

In addition to its nourishment, food is also a reminder of so many ways God supplies us with a plethora of foods and greens and spices that not only are delicious but have the power within them to energize and repair the body. And food is a gift that becomes even more of a blessing when we share it: when we break bread with others or invite them to take a seat at our dinner table. Shared food has the power to unite, create, grow, or restore relationships. And when foods from traditions and cultures other than our own are shared with us, we are educated and our minds are broadened.

In some of the Gospel stories, we see how integral food was to Jesus's relationships with people: food plays an essential role as he helped others, taught others, and fed others and as he demonstrated deeper spiritual meanings through and beyond the food itself.

In those Gospels, we see how Jesus ate with people that the religious leaders refused to associate with. We see how Jesus fed large, hungry crowds, one of five thousand people, even as he offered lessons in abundance. In these interactions we see him teach, educate, share, give, and forgive. The heart of God and the life and service of Jesus are shared from places where food was at the center of the story.

Perhaps one of the most enlightening events of the Bible that revolves around food is the Last Supper—the meal Jesus shared with his closest followers. New Testament scholar N. T. Wright said it best in his book *Simply Jesus* when he shared, "When Jesus himself wanted to explain to his disciples what his forthcoming death was all about, he didn't give them a theory, he gave them a meal."[1]

Today, in our tech-saturated, jam-packed-scheduled, community- and face-to-face-conversation-deprived world, food can offer us a multitude of ways for both the chronically ill and the healthy to share what is good and healing. The dinner table holds so many possibilities: to be the place we rediscover one another, reunite with the people we love, and bring together people who will fall in love as food is shared. It is a place that invites us to open our hearts once again and safely allow ourselves to be vulnerable with others. Over bowls of nourishing soup, we can share our struggles and our victories; over small plates of rugelach, we can admit the challenges we are facing, the prayers we are praying, and the answered prayers we have been blessed through.

Fabulous Finds
New Meal-Time Practices

How can you incorporate a sense of community through new meal-time practices in your home? Perhaps invite new friends over each month, plan a regular potluck night, enact device-free meal zones, or even make a bowl full of questions that people can randomly ask at each meal. There are so many exciting and fun ways to deepen your sense of community with friends and family. Get creative!

Over a meal

- we can break bread with new friends,
- we can look gratefully across the table at family who have been a part of our life since the moment of our birth,
- we can laugh together,
- we can forgive each other,
- we can tell the details of our stories,
- we can cry without judgment,
- we can heal our body, and
- we can experience the love and presence of God.

Today, as I wrote about shared and nourishing food, this overwhelming desire came over me to make a batch of one of my grandmother's favorite desserts—rice pudding. I longed to feel its warm, silky texture on my tongue and taste its hint of cinnamon flavor. As I began to combine the ingredients in the slow cooker, I thought about the ending of this book and how my story couldn't be neatly wrapped up in a bow. There is still so much life to be lived. More challenges to come. More ways to share the lessons I've learned with others. And between the making of the rice pudding and thinking about my grandmother, it got me thinking about all of the individual parts that make up each one of our stories and how some of those parts will carry heavier weight than others.

The heavy weight really gets our attention, and we mistakenly believe that our traumatic events or our illness or our life challenges are the main theme of our story. They're not. Our story isn't about "the sick woman" or "the guy with an immune disorder." We aren't defined by whatever illness or trauma we've experienced.

Within, through, and beyond our story is an even bigger one of faith and overcoming.

When you get that diagnosis or yearlong flare or feel like so much of your life has been ripped away by a sudden event or devastating illness you have little control over, remember your story is a larger, wider one—and it's a story (like food) that nourishes others when shared.

I know my life won't be trial- and challenge-free moving forward. There will be new battles—or familiar ones—around the corner. But I know that from my kitchen view, I have met the healing power of God, the nourishing ingredients I've learned to share, and the memories of my grandmother that promise there's also another answered prayer in the future and a shared dinner table with those I love. I know I can lean on and trust in the support of my mom, Mickey, a loving circle of friends, and the unbelievable community of LupusChick.

So as I curl up on a soft, tufted, oversized chair on my porch, donning black sweats, a fluffy white sweater, and an oversized plaid scarf during a crisp fall evening, I watch the steam rise from the warm vanilla- and cinnamon-infused rice pudding and I think of my grandmother and Jesus and how thankful I am for her sharing her small avocado-green kitchen with me and the teachings from her gentle spirit that showed me the mighty connection between shared food and Jesus—and how both offer healing and nourishment for our lives.

MY PRAYER FOR YOU

You, my friend, are a force to be reckoned with.
You are a mighty warrior beginning to blaze your path through
    an unknown wilderness.
In your valleys, you will rise up.
In your peaks, you will stay humble and kind.

You are unique, and a divine purpose has been poured down
upon you.

You are treasured and loved beyond compare.

You are a million little amazing things that make up your imper-
fectly perfect being.

You are not your illness.

You are not your trauma.

You are the Divine's incredible gift to this world.

And we are so blessed to have you.

Easy Slow Cooker Vanilla Spiced Rice Pudding

Prep Time: 10 minutes
Cook Time: 2.5–3 hours
Method: Stovetop and slow cooker (a 3- or 4-quart slow cooker works well)
Yield: 6 servings

Nothing brings me back to my childhood, my grandmother, and Bogey (my grandfather) quicker than a rich, creamy bowl of rice pudding. With hints of vanilla, cinnamon, a little extra spice thanks to ground cloves, and sweetness from raisins, this dessert may be hard to share! And what makes this dessert even better is that it's incredibly easy—put everything in the slow cooker, make yourself a cup of tea, and go relax. Plus, with substitutions, you can make this dessert dairy-free and with a healthier sugar alternative. Though this recipe is delicious as is, I like to top my rice pudding off with fresh raspberries or raspberry preserves, but you may want to add extra cinnamon or whipped cream (regular or coconut).

INGREDIENTS

1 cup jasmine rice (you can also try arborio or basmati)
⅓ cup butter or butter alternative, melted
4½ cups milk or milk alternative
½ cup granulated sugar or coconut sugar
1½ teaspoons cinnamon
½ teaspoon ground cloves
2 teaspoons vanilla extract
½ cup raisins
Pinch of salt

Optional Toppings

Fresh fruit such as berries
Fruit preserves
Whipped cream
Extra cinnamon

Tips

- For extra creamy rice, swap out ½ cup of liquid for a ½ cup condensed coconut milk.
- I like thick rice pudding, but if you prefer a looser texture, you can add a little extra liquid to it while cooking
- Get creative with flavors—you can add ginger spice, vanilla bean, allspice, caramel, or even rose water.

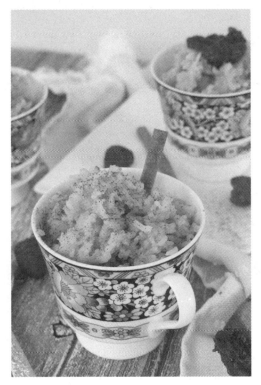

Rinse rice under cold water and drain. Lightly grease your slow cooker with butter or a butter alternative. Melt the ⅓ cup butter or butter alternative and set to the side. Add your rinsed rice, milk, sugar, cinnamon, ground cloves, vanilla extract, raisins, and pinch of salt to the slow cooker. Stir well to combine all the ingredients. Last, pour your melted butter into the slow cooker and stir one last time. Secure the lid on the slow cooker and turn on high. Cook for 2 hours, stir, and check on the rice. Cover and cook for another

15 to 30 minutes, checking often, until all the liquid has been absorbed. Depending on the slow cooker, the rice pudding may be fully cooked at the 2-hour mark or 2.5-hour mark or may take longer. Just pop it open every so often, give it a stir, and see if the consistency is to your liking. Serve immediately in small bowls, add desired toppings, and enjoy! I prefer to serve this right away, as this rice pudding tends to get thick, especially when refrigerated.

Notes

CHAPTER 2

1. "9 Scientifically Proven Reasons to Eat Dinner as a Family," Goodnet, May 5, 2016, https://tinyurl.com/y4rpbe5q.

CHAPTER 3

1. Megan E. Speer, Jamil P. Bhanji, and Mauricio R. Delgado, "Savoring the Past: Positive Memories Evoke Value Representations in the Striatum," *Neuron* 84, no. 4 (November 19, 2014): 847–56, https://tinyurl.com/y3h94coj.
2. Maria Konnikova, "Why We Need Answers," *New Yorker*, 2017, accessed December 31, 2019, https://tinyurl.com/y3dqqmg6; Arie Kruglanski and Donna Webster, "Individual Difference in Need for Cognitive Closure," *Journal of Personality and Social Psychology* 67, no. 6 (January 1995): 1049–62, accessed December 31, 2019, https://tinyurl.com/y2gmwdn4; Arie Kruglanski and Shira Fishman, "The Need for Cognitive Closure," American Psychological Association, 2009, accessed December 31, 2019, https://tinyurl.com/y4w9uk8h.

CHAPTER 4

1. Imke Kirste, "Is Silence Golden? Effects of Auditory Stimuli and Their Absence on Adult Hippocampal Neurogenesis," *Brain Structure and Function*, December 2013, accessed December 31, 2019, https://tinyurl.com/yyz59n9f.
2. L. Bernardi, "Cardiovascular, Cerebrovascular, and Respiratory Changes Induced by Different Types of Music in Musicians and Non-musicians: The Importance of Silence," *Heart* 92,

no. 4 (December 9, 2005): 445–52, accessed April 28, 2019, https://tinyurl.com/y2of3zqx.

3. Hamed Ekhtiari and Martin Paulus, eds., *Neuroscience for Addiction Medicine: From Prevention to Rehabilitation—Constructs and Drugs*, Progress in Brain Research (Amsterdam: Elsevier, 2016), https://tinyurl.com/y2wja2c3; Michael D. Greicius, Ben Krasnow, Allan L. Reiss, and Vinod Menon, "Functional Connectivity in the Resting Brain: A Network Analysis of the Default Mode Hypothesis," *Proceedings of the National Academy of Sciences USA* 100, no. 1 (January 7, 2003): 253–58, https://tinyurl.com/y2cerknm.

4. T. D. Jakes (@BishopJakes), "The reward you get for overcoming your last challenge is your next challenge," Twitter, July 12, 2019, https://tinyurl.com/y38x94lb.

5. "Autoimmune Diseases," National Institute of Environmental Health Sciences, accessed November 25, 2020, https://tinyurl.com/yylmvho4.

6. "Our Mission," American Autoimmune Related Diseases Association, accessed November 6, 2020, https://www.aarda.org/who-we-are/.

CHAPTER 5

1. See Carmen Ambrosio, *Life Continues: Facing the Challenges of MS, Menopause and Midlife with Hope, Courage and Humor* (Dublin, OH: AMBROSart, 2010).

2. Kendra Cherry, "Locus of Control and Your Life," Verywell Mind, December 7, 2019, https://tinyurl.com/yxjuwrnd.

3. Emily Sutherlin, "Autoimmune Diseases: Why Our Body Sometimes Turns on Itself," Genetic Literacy Project, January 12, 2018, https://tinyurl.com/y6rktm7y/; Ana-Maria Orbai, "Autoimmune Disease: Why Is My Immune System Attacking Itself?," Hopkins Medicine, 2019, accessed January 2, 2020, https://tinyurl.com/yy9kxzvy.

4. "What Causes Lupus?," Lupus Foundation of America, 2018, accessed January 3, 2020, http://www.lupus.org/resources/what-causes-lupus.

5. "Autoimmune Diseases and Their Possible Environmental Triggers," Hospital for Special Surgery, 2012, accessed January 3, 2020, https://tinyurl.com/y5aohu6k.
6. "Autoimmune Diseases," National Institute of Environmental Health Sciences, 2018, accessed January 3, 2020, https://tinyurl.com/y42h79pg.
7. "Autoimmune Diseases."
8. "What Causes Lupus?"
9. "Autoimmune Disease List," American Autoimmune Related Diseases Association, 2017, accessed January 3, 2020, http://www.aarda.org/diseaselist/.
10. "Diagnosing Autoimmune Diseases," Benaroya Research Institute, October 20, 2017, accessed January 3, 2020, https://tinyurl.com/yygvnwds.
11. "Lupus Facts and Statistics," Lupus Foundation of America, 2018, accessed January 3, 2020, https://tinyurl.com/y3zld9ox.
12. Siobhan Fenton, "How Sexist Stereotypes Mean Doctors Ignore Women's Pain," *Independent*, July 27, 2016, accessed January 3, 2020, https://tinyurl.com/y3xcnpd4; Elizabeth G. Nabel, "Coronary Heart Disease in Women—an Ounce of Prevention," *New England Journal of Medicine* 343, no. 8 (August 24, 2000): 572–74.
13. "Policy of Inclusion of Women in Clinical Trials," Womenshealth.gov, August 15, 2017, accessed January 3, 2020, http://www.womenshealth.gov/30-achievements/04; "NIH Policy and Guidelines on the Inclusion of Women and Minorities as Subjects in Clinical Research," NIH.gov, 2019, accessed January 3, 2020, https://tinyurl.com/y38pqfr8.
14. "The Myth of Female Hysteria and Health Disparities among Women," RTI International, May 9, 2018, accessed January 3, 2020, https://tinyurl.com/y6h4odqm.
15. Camille Noe Pagán, "When Doctors Downplay Women's Health Concerns," *New York Times*, May 3, 2018, accessed January 3, 2020, https://tinyurl.com/y3xnlsy4; Gabrielle Levy, "Dying to Be Heard," *US News & World Report*, 2018, accessed January 4,

2020, https://tinyurl.com/y3dhaxhk; Pat Anson, "Women in Pain Report Significant Gender Bias," *National Pain Report*, September 12, 2014, accessed January 3, 2020, https://tinyurl.com/w6awj2p.

CHAPTER 6

1. Joni Eareckson Tada, "Reflections on the 50th Anniversary of My Diving Accident," Gospel Coalition, July 30, 2017, accessed January 4, 2020, https://tinyurl.com/y2qudhm2.

CHAPTER 7

1. See Leen Oris et al., "Illness Identity in Adults with a Chronic Illness," *Journal of Clinical Psychology in Medical Settings* 25, no. 4 (December 2018): 429–40, https://pubmed.ncbi.nlm.nih.gov/29468569/; and Liesbet Van Bulck, Eva Goossens, Koen Luyckx, Leen Oris, Silke Apers, and Philip Moons, "Illness Identity: A Novel Predictor for Healthcare Use in Adults with Congenital Heart Disease," *Journal of the American Heart Association*, May 22, 2018, https://tinyurl.com/y3nybx8a.

CHAPTER 12

1. "NIH Scientists Find Link between Allergic and Autoimmune Diseases in Mouse Study," NIH, June 2, 2013, https://tinyurl.com/y6fskqls; "Allergies & Autoimmune Disease," AHN, accessed November 6, 2020, https://tinyurl.com/y6t8nthx; "Food Allergens May Trigger Development of Autoimmune Diseases, Other Food Allergic Diseases," UNC Health, June 26, 2019, https://tinyurl.com/y5b3qp55.

CHAPTER 14

1. See N. T. Wright, *Simply Jesus* (New York: HarperOne, 2011).